The Best-Laid Plans
Health Care's Problems and Prospects

The Best-Laid Plans

Health Care's Problems and Prospects

LAWRIE MCFARLANE
AND CARLOS PRADO

McGill-Queen's University Press
Montreal & Kingston · London · Ithaca

© McGill-Queen's University Press 2002
ISBN 0-7735-2364-2 (cloth)
ISBN 0-7735-2365-0 (paper)

Legal deposit second quarter 2002
Bibliothèque nationale du Québec

Printed in Canada on acid-free paper

McGill-Queen's University Press acknowledges the
financial support of the Government of Canada
through the Book Publishing Industry Development
Program (BPIDP) for its publishing activities. We also
acknowledge the support of the Canada Council for
the Arts for our publishing program.

National Library of Canada Cataloguing
in Publication Data

McFarlane, Lawrie
    The best-laid plans: health care's problems
    and prospects
    Includes bibliographical references and index.
    ISBN 0-7735-2364-2 (bound). –
    ISBN 0-7735-2365-0 (pbk.)
    1. Health care reform – Canada. 2. Medical care –
    Canada. I. Prado, C.G. II. Title.
    RA395.C3M39 2002   362.1'0971   C2001-903517-9

Typeset in Palatino 10/13
by Caractéra inc., Quebec City

For Anne and Catherine

Contents

Foreword

As we begin the twenty-first century, "medicare" is a defining characteristic of being Canadian, although most would be hard pressed to define it even in general terms. It is our most cherished – and single most expensive – social program. Repeated public opinion polls show that medicare's preservation, indeed its expansion and enhancement, is in a class by itself among government expenditures for which people seem prepared to pay more rather than less in taxes. There is a strong commitment to share publicly the financial risk of disease and injury – risk that, before medicare, was borne alone by those affected, their families, and those who would extend them charity. This commitment is widely shared from coast to coast and is a tribute to the coherence and underlying goodness of contemporary Canadian society.

Yet medicare, shorthand for Canada's health care system, is not what it seems. At best it is ten provincial and three territorial programs that use public money to insure people against the costs of hospital and physicians' services, loosely coordinated by virtue of their common adherence, more or less, to the five principles of the Canada Health Act of 1984. At worst, there is no *system*, using the word in its ordinary sense to mean a collection of interrelated components or parts (physicians, hospitals, pharmacies, home care, etc.) acting together synergistically so both quality and productivity are greater than when each acts independently.

This book makes the case that there is not now, nor can there ever be, a genuine health care system. Neither can there be continuity of care, because health care is unmanageable; at least it cannot be managed centrally or on a macro scale. The case is set out theoretically by application to health care of genealogical and ethical analyses developed by Michel Foucault, analyses primarily developed from studies of the effects on people of institutional practices and vice versa. These analyses support the conclusion that planning and management are not possible in the complex ("chaotic") institution of health care, primarily because the behaviours of those affected, whether agents or clients, cannot be predicted. The theoretical framework is filled in by an examination of actual management decisions taken by successive federal and provincial governments over the past twenty years as they have struggled in vain to produce and apply a viable management model for the delivery of health care services.

Although it remains that most people who have sought and used hospital and physicians' services throughout Canada agree that they have been well served, most informed observers agree that medicare is a mess. It is beset by many problems, most of them of long-standing and worsening. There is a strong consensus among Canadians, however, that medicare should remain a public program, indeed that the publicly insured services provided should be expanded to include prescription drugs and home care especially, as well as long-term care, which also claims priority for many.

To meet people's growing expectations within a public system for universal, accessible, portable, comprehensive services of high quality requires that the providers – physicians, hospitals, nurses, nursing homes, home care, pharmacists, and so on – coordinate their work to meet the particular needs of their individual patients/clients/customers and their families and communities. In other words, they must conform to the discipline of a system with a clearly defined vision and mission, with explicit goals, objectives, and policies that create the incentives necessary to channel individual self-interests and hold them accountable to serve the common good. Where such systemization really counts, however, is at the workface, the level where the providers and consumers (and prospective consumers) of health care themselves have a stake in the outcomes of greater synergy – increased productivity and higher quality services throughout the continuum of care. Elsewhere the purposes are principally bureaucratic and the results too often, as the authors point out, counterproductive.

Why is it so difficult to build a genuine system of health care services? The four principal roadblocks are:

• Our governments shrink from governing; they avoid providing the leadership every system requires. They persist in the delusion that health services should and can be managed at a distance from the consumers and providers affected. This book focuses on the theoretical and experiential reasons that solving medicare's problems through "better management" is not now working and will not work in future.

- There are no clear lines of accountability between the public and the providers, managers, and the (absent) governors of medicare.
- Entrenched interests create the perception that even discussion of change in medicare is the political equivalent of the "third rail." Resistance to change by those interests and their capacity to incite the media to fearmongering are problems of major proportion.
- No province or territory has the capacity for effective health information management.

From their two perspectives, theory and praxis, the authors provide an interesting and provocative analysis of the etiology of medicare's ills, and a diagnosis of what is really wrong. Surprisingly, given the blame attached to and issue taken with health reform's mavens, the recommended approach to treatment is not far off what I and many others believe necessary to make medicare work for the benefit of Canada's communities and population into the twenty-first century.[1]

Duncan G. Sinclair
Chair of the former Health Services
Restructuring Commission (Ontario) and
Visiting Fellow, School of Policy Studies,
Queen's University at Kingston

Preface

Health Care Services and/or Disease Management

Sometime in the last century, the bright new words "health care services" crept into our Canadian vocabulary to replace the more paternalistic and gloomy implications conveyed by older formulas involving "medicine," "doctors," and "hospitals." Euphemism? Perhaps. But the shift in vocabulary reflects several realities: workers in the field include nurses, physiotherapists, social workers, and teachers, as well as physicians and surgeons; many people who apply for help are not actually sick; and hospitals are not always the locus of activity. More recently, and in keeping with the trend, "patients" have become "clients" or "consumers," while "workers" are known as "providers" or members of "teams." The language of efficient business management is ascendant. Riding on its coattails is the vanguard of evidence-based medicine, which relies on randomized controlled trials to generate guidelines for practice that ought to have wide applicability for all peoples even as they innocently (and erroneously) imply that the medicine of the past was based on little or no evidence at all. These changes have prompted a "managerial" response to the provision, administration, and periodic reform of health care.

As attractive and reasonable as the semantic change may be, the system itself is said to be in crisis. Constraints on funding are often cited as the cause of the crisis, but McFarlane and Prado demonstrate that the funding issues are only one symptom of deeper social and philosophical problems. The concept of "Health Care Services" ignores certain other realities of our so-called health care system, and, indeed, the shift in nomenclature proclaims a fundamental conceptual problem at the root of the current crisis.

For example, if these "services" are to be run on a market model of supply and demand, which is amenable to business management concepts, then we should have a clear idea of their product: "health." But the definition of health is slippery and individualistic. It has challenged generations of scholars who, in exasperation, resort to defining it as the lack of its apparent opposite, disease. The oft-cited definition used by the World Health Organization tries to avoid this problem by investing health with positive attributes, not just the absence of disease. Health is defined as a state of physical, mental, and social well-being. But whatever positive attributes "health" may enjoy, it must not include disease. The task of health care services becomes clear and simple when it fixes on this common denominator: the "services" are predicated on treating, identifying, or preventing disease, whether or not the product is health. Their success is charted, even by the World Health Organization, in statistics on morbidity, mortality, and elimination of disease. To qualify for "health care services," the "client" must present through a disease rubric and with potential disease in mind. Despite the lip service paid to the social determinants of health – education, literacy, employment, wealth, personal autonomy, and political freedom – we do not offer health care services in our current system; we offer disease management and prevention.

For at least fifty years, historians and philosophers have shown that disease concepts are ideas that are socially constructed, related to cultural norms as well as individual biological functions. If social values enter into what we classify as "sick," they also enter into what we classify as "healthy." Analysis of the hidden messages in public- and private-sector health information shows that images of health are inadvertently young, able-bodied, thin, white, and middle-class. We know, however, that the elderly, the poor, and the disabled can be healthy within their own frames of reference. In fact, each person should reasonably be the best judge of the state of his or her own health.

Since the middle of the nineteenth century, however, most educated people concede some power in that decision to the judgment of a physician. They know that the stethoscope, the blood pressure cuff, the blood test, the urinalysis, the Pap smear, the X-ray, and scanners can detect traces of disease long before symptoms are felt. And early detection, we believe, is a good way to prevent devastating illness. Immunization is another. Without diminishing the crucial role of medical and surgical treatments, reassurance is a huge part of what should be meant by "care," both for those who are dying and for those without symptoms who display entirely normal results following investigations. Care must include recognition of the vulnerability and dependence of the "client" upon personal contact with an expert.

But what about "care" in our so-called health care system? How is caring a management model? Even if treatment is not working, even if normal tests fail to assuage fears, must we dismiss the individual by a Tayloristic[1] formula that proscribes further investment in her problem? In a privileged society such as ours, does not everyone have the right to speedy attention and sympathetic concern, an ear to listen, a hand to hold? Are these old-fashioned notions associated with traditional nursing and medicine no longer worthy of public resources? And can a collectivity of bureaucrats or insurance providers using population-based statistics determine how much care is appropriate for each problem, when – as we have already seen – the so-called "health" problems are as myriad as individual personalities and life experiences? Are we prepared to allow the private sector to determine premiums for a caregiving that will hold just the right number of hands and preserve life for just the right number of years, while it also yields a profit to the insurance industry? Programmatic definitions of health care needs are impossible because they seek to impose a uniform order on chaotic perceptions of health, a chaos that we should honour and celebrate. Little wonder that the various guidelines generated for disease management and prevention are lauded more than they are used.

In sum, our health care system forces individuals to cede power to experts whom they must approach through a disease-based system. Far from accepting that health and health needs are concepts as widely diverse as the peoples of our land, we try to ignore the domination of disease and pretend that health is a non-controversial, material commodity to be meted out in rationalized allotments by managers. Money is neither the biggest nor the only problem. As McFarlane and Prado show, illusion and misunderstanding contribute to the reasons that our health care system is sick; more important, attempts to fix the system that are based on managerial assumptions ignore these intrinsic reasons for its problems.

Jacalyn M. Duffin, MD, FRCP (C)
Hannah Chair, History of Medicine,
Queen's University

The Best-Laid Plans

Introduction

Medicare is the operational system by which Canadians receive essential health services. It embodies certain obligations and confers certain entitlements. Widely believed to be one of the defining accomplishments of our nationhood, medicare has grown, in less than forty years, from a distant objective to a present entitlement of all Canadians.

This book was written because the authors believe that medicare is imperilled to a significant degree, for reasons largely unknown to most Canadians. Few would disagree that something is seriously amiss with health care in Canada. However, that consensus is matched by another that we think is wrong-headed. This second consensus is that the way to fix whatever is wrong with health care is with more funding and better macro-level management. Certainly more funding would fix many things that are wrong, but not only are there limits to available funding, just throwing money at health care will not fix everything. It is a mistake to think that health care's problems are all of the sort that can be resolved either with more funding and/or better management. It is the burden of this book to say how this is the case, and to suggest what might be done to properly address the health care crisis.

We approach health care's crisis from very different perspectives, but we both believe strongly that the nature of health care's problems, and in fact the nature of health care itself, is misperceived by those who think its problems can be effectively addressed with current management techniques. Assuming limited funding, health care's problems are of two sorts: the kind that is amenable to being solved or improved with better management and the kind that is not so amenable because it is inherent in health care itself. It is this latter sort of problem that accounts for the recurrent nature of the crisis, and that forms the subject matter of our inquiry.

Though our conclusions about the nature of health care's present difficulties coincide, the ways we each have reached those conclusions are different. In what follows, then, there are two voices. We believe this is to the good, because we are able to present a clearer picture of what has gone wrong with health care and attempts to reform it.

For one of us (Prado), health care's problems pose a series of conceptual questions. These questions have to do with the nature of hierarchical and structured human interaction. That is, they essentially have to do with who we think we are and how we act when we engage with others in managed activity. Though they admit of varying articulation, I have put these questions as follows: How do large-scale enterprises, such as health care, work – and fail to work – as they do? Are there principles or even rough guidelines to help us understand why carefully planned and implemented large-scale enterprises so often produce unanticipated and usually unwelcome results? Why is it that when sizable numbers of people jointly strive to achieve certain ends, what they actually achieve frequently is counter to their objectives? Is it because there is something inherently problematic about large-scale managed activity involving hierarchical structure, administration, and supervision? Does something happen to people who become involved in such activity that makes them act in unexpected ways? Are people who engage in managed large-scale enterprises affected by what others do in special, behaviour-determining ways? Is each of us somehow a different person when subjected to management? How is each of us shaped and moulded to be the persons we become in the context of an enterprise that involves management of our activity?

For the other of us (McFarlane), the recurrence of the health care crisis raises some fundamental questions about how governments have tried to manage health care. These questions have a personal aspect. As the CEO of a regional health authority in Saskatchewan, and later as deputy minister of health in British Columbia, I saw firsthand the efforts made by provincial governments to implement health reform. If political courage, expert advisers, and sheer hard work were sufficient, the management problems in health care would have been solved by now. Instead, it appears that the reform programs have not succeeded, and indeed may actually have exacerbated the problems. Yet these initiatives were not simply tinkering or fine-tuning; they involved the wholesale adoption of a completely new management model of health delivery. If we now accept that this model has failed, then a major part of the conceptual framework within which the provinces manage health care must also be jettisoned and a new approach found.

In the first part of this book, we explore how health care poses problems that elude current management thinking. We draw attention to some fundamental characteristics of human behaviour, particularly in institutional settings, and show how these limit the enterprise of managing in ways not understood by health care reform advocates.

The first four chapters are devoted to the questions about hierarchical, structured human interaction. In chapter 1, we consider some ideas that clarify how institutions and individuals define one another. In chapter 2, we consider how those ideas apply to health care. In chapter 3, we look at parallels between health care and what are called "chaotic dynamical systems." In chapter 4, we offer a summation of the major points presented in the first three.

In the second part, we use these insights to illustrate how, and why, the standard health care reform program has failed; we also draw attention to inherent flaws in the privatization alternative.

In chapter 5, we chart the historical origins of the crisis in health care, including the succession of efforts to manage the crisis. In chapter 6, we look more closely at the various prescriptions that the orthodox reform approach has employed to regain control of medicare. This leads us to a more detailed examination, in chapter 7, of the internal dynamics of medicare. In chapters 8 and 9, we clarify the nature of our entitlement, as citizens, to health care, and in chapter 10, we examine the privatization alternative, which the government of Alberta has proposed. Finally, in chapter 11, we propose a new approach to managing health care delivery in Canada, consistent with the conceptual base we have developed.

We are aware of the radical nature of our critique: if we are right, much political capital and fifteen years of heartbreaking management effort have been expended in vain. We believe that the failure of health care reform to meet its stated goals and, in particular, to restore financial sustainability to medicare entitles us to a hearing. We believe that medicare can be saved, but only at the cost of adopting a solution that, in the present state of health policy thinking, must appear heretical: this is that medicare needs less managing, not more.

PART ONE

Some Theory

CHAPTER ONE

Health Care and Our Theoretical Base

Robert Burns warned that our best-laid plans often go awry, and Murphy's Law holds that if anything can go wrong, it will. It is a hard fact of life that our endeavours are plagued by unexpected and undesired results, even when we avoid making mistakes. This is especially true when those endeavours involve large numbers of people, and nowhere is this more evident than in health care's management, periodic reforms, and recent history.

The frequency with which health care policies and management have yielded unexpected and undesired results suggests that the reasons usually given for why things go wrong do not explain what actually does go wrong. Otherwise, efforts to fix health care should have had positive results by now. Instead, efforts to reform health care in various ways and to various degrees have failed to improve health care and in some cases have even worsened its delivery. We think the reasons for health care's problems, and for its worrying prospects, are inadequately understood. And if the reasons that reform is needed in the first place are not fully understood, efforts to reform health care are likely to continue to prove ineffective or counterproductive.

The list of the usual things on which policy and delivery debacles and derailments are normally blamed is a longish one, and it is not exhaustive. Some of the most common items are:

- Bad planning
- Distorted or deficient data
- Inadequate funding
- Administrative error

- Unforeseen developments
- Inept or misguided assessments
- Recalcitrant bureaucracies
- Vested interests
- Systemic biases
- Gender issues
- Incompetence
- Corruption
- Deliberate partisan sabotage

Unquestionably, these factors play their parts in policy implementation and delivery going wrong, and unfortunately none of them can be wholly eliminated. But we may be missing something important if we are content to blame only these factors, and others like them, when things go amiss. These factors cause confusion; they plague the setting up and running of anything from a corner store to a multinational corporation. These factors are basically various kinds of misjudgments; ignorance; knowing, factional, or self-serving actions; and inadvertent or intentional obstructionist behaviour. As such, these factors are inherent in all human activity. People inevitably make mistakes, have limited knowledge, act self-interestedly, and innocently or deliberately thwart others' efforts. What we need to consider about health care's problems is that more is going on than the usual and inevitable slip-ups and missteps. We have to consider that things go wrong with health care because of something intrinsic to the enterprise itself. That is, we have to consider whether there is not something about the large-scale management and delivery of health care that generates problems peculiar to the enterprise.

To consistently blame health care's problems and failures on the range of perennial human errors that beleaguer all of our endeavours is to assume that when something goes wrong, it is because something else was overlooked, misdescribed, misconstrued, not anticipated and allowed for in planning, misapplied, not adhered to, misunderstood, or circumvented in practice. To think this way is to consider health care and its management too mechanistically; it is to see problems and failures as solely due to design or operational flaws. This view seems to be an integral element in current business-model thinking about the initiation and management of enterprises. Widespread application of this thinking to health care means that there is a strong tendency to neglect the possibility that health care's problems are due not only to bad design or execution, but also to something intrinsic to health care itself.

We believe that health care, as an enterprise, is special, even unique, in the degree or extent of its complexity and diverse characteristics. We also believe that our account of the nature of health care's complexity is original in that it brings together a number of factors that for too long have been considered in isolation. The key point is that, aside from its management and delivery being impeded by the sorts of extrinsic disruptive factors listed above, health care generates a variety of its own problems. Health care is special because of two different but tightly integrated elements that define it as an enterprise. The first element that makes health care special is that health care changes its agents and clients.[1] That is, health care affects the people who manage and deliver it, as well as the people it serves, in ways that significantly alter their self-images, attitudes, and behaviour. While any activity engaged in for long enough has its effects on its agents and clients, managing, delivering, and receiving health care does so in especially profound ways. To understand how and why this is the case, it has to be appreciated that not only does health care affect people's well-being and their very lives, it is as much an institution as are education and the military. In other words, health care is a structured whole that, in the process of fulfilling its purpose, organizes and regulates people's conduct, time, and physical location. Health care requires certain behaviour from both its practitioners and patients, it imposes schedules on them, and it locates them in particular places – hospitals, clinics, doctors' offices, diagnostic labs, and so on. While it may be obvious that health care affects people's lives in profound ways, what is less obvious, and concerns us most, is that by affecting people as it does, health care directly and indirectly causes them to behave in ways that in turn affect health care in unexpected and often negative ways. In order to understand how health care changes its agents and clients, and how in turn their behaviour changes health care, we need to establish a theoretical base and introduce some special terminology. That is what we attempt to do in this chapter.

The second element that makes health care special is its complexity. Health care's complexity is of a very high order. This complexity includes the variety and extent of health care's physical resources and the circumstances of the sites in which it is practised. Health care's complexity also includes the volatility of the policies that govern it, the convolutions of the social contexts in which it is conducted, and especially the intricacies of the interactions among its agents and clients. To better understand health care's complexity, we have to look hard at that complexity from two different perspectives. One focuses specifically on human interactions, while the other focuses on health care's similarities to other complex systems. In the next chapter we consider how the behaviour of health care's agents and clients is partly determined by random consequences of their interactions. In chapter 3, we consider how health care's unpredictability is a special case of systemic unpredictability, and how its agents and clients increase its unpredictability through efforts at self-determination. Chapter 4 provides a summary of the main points considered in the first three chapters. Our aim in chapters 1, 2, 3, and 4 is to provide a productive theoretical context and base for what follows in subsequent chapters.

HEALTH CARE AS AN INSTITUTION

We begin by stressing that health care is an institution; it is an institution in the way education, the military, and the judicial and penal systems are institutions. Like other institutions, health care affects and, to an extent, controls people's lives. And, like other institutions, health care affects and controls people's lives in ways that have repercussions to how it itself functions and succeeds or fails. The Canadian health care institution is in crisis. Its cost seems to be increasingly unmanageable, and efforts to control costs have resulted in such things as jammed emergency rooms and long waits for surgery; as a consequence, its universality is being challenged. Most people who are concerned with reforming health care to resolve its crisis seem to think that what is wrong can be fixed with policy and management changes. We contend that health care poses special problems that are not due to the extrinsic factors usually blamed for things going wrong, so policy and management changes of the sort envisaged will fix little or nothing, and may, in fact, make matters worse. Health care's special problems differ from those that can be dealt with by tinkering with policy and management, because those problems are not caused by extrinsic factors that are amenable to that sort of adjustment or remedy. Some of health care's special problems have to do with how health care alters the perceptions and self-images of those who provide it and those who receive it. The heart of the trouble is that, in altering perceptions and self-images, health care prompts unpredictable behaviour.

Delivering or receiving medical care inevitably influences how individuals see themselves, their situations, and their prospects. How health care is managed has crucial consequences for how practitioners see themselves and their roles, and how they practise medicine; how health care is managed also has crucial consequences for how patients see themselves and their roles, and how they receive treatment. Health care is delivered and received in ways structured and regulated by management policies and practices; the impact on agents and clients alike is inescapable. Management's impact on practitioners and patients is all the more consequential because of the value-laden nature of medical policies and objectives, the emotional content of medical decisions, and the vulnerability of those needing care. But when we say that health care changes its agents and clients, its practitioners and patients, it is important to understand that the changes in question go beyond such things as a physician becoming cynical or a patient becoming fatalistic. The changes are about *who one is* in the context of health care, and that determines how one acts in that context.

As noted, the key to understanding why health care generates particularly troublesome issues is appreciating that in changing its agents and clients, health care makes their behaviour unpredictable. Health care's agents and clients are like molecular components that act differently when combined than when isolated. That sort of unpredictability prevents effective anticipation of how implementing a policy or changing a management practice will work out. For reasons we consider in detail below, we cannot determine what the functioning institution of health care will look like at some point in the future by simply inventorying its components and surveying how they have behaved in the past. This is the great weakness of excessive reliance on statistical models. Health care management, like all contemporary types of management, relies heavily on statistics-based assessments and projections to configure and organize its services and procedures. But if the activities of health care's agents and clients are structured and regulated in ways that inadvertently transform how they see themselves, health care, their place in it, and their obligations and entitlements, their behaviour will not conform to the statistical models. Predictions based on statistical models are only as good as the stability of what the models portray. Statistics-based predictions and projections are attempts at determining the sort of working institution that will result from changing or combining certain components in certain ways. But if the components in question are not stable, if they behave unexpectedly when changed or combined, the predictions and projections will prove to be of little use. Few enterprises can continue to function smoothly when their agents and clients begin to act differently from how planners and managers intend and expect them to act. Matters are worsened when reforms are instituted, because agents and clients, who have adjusted to one set of policies and practices, then have to deal with new sets. That leads to confusion, increased resistance to change, and the risk that some old ways of doing things will continue despite lip service to the new ways.

We believe that there has been far too little attention paid to how health care affects its agents and clients as individuals, and to how the resulting behaviour of those agents and clients impairs or even vitiates health care's objectives. We want to clarify how health care affects its agents and clients in ways that change those agents and clients and makes them behave in unpredictable ways. We also want to say a good deal about health care itself, and past and proposed changes to it, to clarify how and why things have gone wrong and what might be done to improve matters.

To achieve the first objective, saying how health care changes its people, we apply – and somewhat extend – some of Michel Foucault's "genealogical" and "ethical" analytic ideas.[2] Much of Foucault's genealogical work concerns how institutional regulation and what he calls "discipline" change people by changing their behaviour and so their self-images, attitudes, and values.[3] Foucault's ethical work concerns not individuals' obligations to others, as one would expect, but individuals' relations to themselves, and especially how people change themselves in the process of trying to be the persons they want to be.

Foucauldian genealogy is a mode of analysis that uses meticulous empirical research to ground the retelling of an institution's history. And the sense of "institution" is broad; along with genealogical analyses of the asylum, the clinic, and the penitentiary, Foucault offers a genealogical analysis of nothing less than human sexuality. However, our aims are more modest. Though initially it may seem odd, for our purposes it is genealogical analysis of the penal system that is most relevant to our analysis of health care. It is in his treatment of penality that we find Foucault's most pertinent insights into how institutions function. It is in that treatment that his earlier analyses of the asylum and clinic have their fruition and are articulated in terms that apply to any institution that manages large numbers of people with a view to delivering an essential service.

Foucault's strategy is to highlight and connect previously marginal and obscured elements and events to present a new developmental picture of the targeted institution, a picture very different from the one the institution itself presents or the one that is presented by traditional historians. The aim is to better understand "the objectivizing of the subject."[4] This is how individuals are objectified and shaped by an institution's regulations and practices through having their behaviour regulated, their status defined, and themselves inculcated with certain values and self-images. Mapping of what Foucault calls "power relations," or simply "power," is the heart of genealogical analysis. "Power" or "power relations" are not overt or even covert force or coercion, as it is natural to assume. Power or power relations are how the totality of people's complexly interrelated activities bear on what each one does. Our extension of Foucault's ideas involves considering how the individuals that an institution controls in turn affect that institution. This extension of genealogy involves application of Foucauldian ethical views, which have to do with "the way a human being turns him– or herself into a subject."[5] The extension allows us to show how health care's agents and clients redefine themselves and how, in doing so, they act in ways that affect the health care management policies and techniques that regulate their behaviour and imbue them with values and images of themselves.[6]

A crucially important point about both Foucault's genealogical and his ethical ideas is how he conceives of subjects. He uses the term "subject," particularly in his genealogical work, in a deliberately compound sense to capture how each of us is both a *conscious subject* and a *governed subject*. That is, each of us is a self-aware being and a being whose activities are regulated by institutions, the state, and society at large. In genealogy, the emphasis is on how institutional disciplines define governed subjects, and Foucault casts the self-aware subject as a product of the way the governed subject is controlled. In ethics, Foucault emphasizes how self-aware subjects govern and so define themselves. The importance of this duality is that though individuals may be defined as subjects by institutional and social control, each has a particular history and responds to being governed in ways dictated by that history. In addition, each is trying to become a particular subject or kind of subject. This means that the control that institutions exert on individuals is exerted on people who are protean, who are

continuously adapting to a multitude of external and internal influences. This malleability, this plasticity, is at the heart of our claim that
some of health care's problems are due to reasons peculiar to it and
to how it changes its agents and clients.

In connection with the malleability of subjects, we need to note
that Foucault was strangely silent on an aspect of human relations
that concerns us greatly in our time. That aspect is gender. As will
be evident in what follows, especially in several of the examples we
use, gender is a crucial element in how health care works and fails
to work as an institution. Foucault's silence on gender, a silence for
which he has been widely criticized, seems to have had to do in part
with his own sexual orientation, and in part with his likely believing
that gender issues are too much a part of the "deployed" or socially
constructed sexuality he exposed in the first volume of *The History of
Sexuality*.[7] This is an important limiting factor in Foucault's analytic
framework, given the importance of gender in the investigation of
health care's problems and prospects.

We now need to discuss Foucauldian genealogy and ethics enough
to provide a productive theoretical perspective on the discussion of
health care that follows in subsequent chapters.

OUR THEORETICAL BASE

Richard Rorty contends that Foucault's most important contribution
is showing how "patterns of acculturation" impose on contemporary
society's members "constraints of which older, premodern societies
had not dreamed."[8] What Rorty is referring to is how institutions and
society at large shape people, not only through prescriptive and
proscriptive rules and enforcement, but also by inculcating *norms*.
Foucault shows us how inculcation of norms is a far more effective
device for controlling people than are dictates, threats, and brute
force. In his major genealogical works, *Discipline and Punish* and the
first volume of *The History of Sexuality*, Foucault describes how institutional disciplinary techniques shape the individuals they control,
less by forcing them to behave in specified ways than by "normalizing" them. That is, rather than merely forcing unwilling compliance
with rules and regulations, modern institutions and societies achieve
compliance by effecting changes in people through getting them to
internalize promoted standards, values, construals, and self-images.
This bears directly on health care and its failures. Health care is an

institution, in Foucault's sense as well as the ordinary sense. It manages large numbers of agents and clients by structuring and regulating their behaviour and, in the process, imbuing them with promoted standards and objectives and, most important, certain images of themselves as providers and recipients of health care. Examples of how this actually works are legion, running from how practitioners are dealt with in medical school to how they are overseen in their residency to how they are initiated into the routines of particular hospitals and wards. On the patient side, examples are even more obvious, running from how they are dealt with during diagnosis and testing to the rituals of hospital admission to how their afflictions are described to them to what they are told and not told. Moreover, gender, race, age, and economic class condition all of this management, so that the actual application of management varies in many ways depending on the gender, race, age, and economic circumstances of those doing the managing and those managed. Health care's agents and clients, then, are all complexly disciplined subjects, regardless of their status or level of responsibility. A standard thesaurus gives "instruct" and "regulate" as synonyms for "discipline," and like soldiers or schoolchildren, health care's agents and clients are instructed and regulated in being practitioners and patients.

What tends to be overlooked, though, is that while institutions change both the people who serve them and the people they serve, there is a reciprocal change effected on the institutions. Changes brought about in agents and clients, as a consequence of discipline, instruction, and regulation, in turn have their effects on their institutions. The way this works is complicated. First of all, in the case of health care, managing it means doing a number of things, such as implementing budgetary policies and imposing directives on practitioners. What managers do determines how individuals conduct themselves as health care providers, such as practitioners not scheduling some expensive tests for patients that they might otherwise have scheduled. What managers do also determines how individuals conduct themselves as health care recipients, such as acquiescing to longer waiting periods for tests or surgery. At this first level, the actions of some constrain the actions of others in a fairly straightforward way. At a second level, constraints are more complex. Health care's agents and clients do the things they do in certain ways, thereby weaving a network of interconnected actions that expands the scope of their more straightforward responses to management directives. This happens because directives always are interpreted and enacted in particular situations. Two hospitals in the same municipality, and two wards in the same hospital, will comply with various directives in different ways or "styles." How things are done in particular contexts evolves as part of a more general working ethos. The result is that the things managers do, and the things practitioners and patients do, interrelate in somewhat different ways because of local conditions. This locally conditioned character of interaction generates a third level at which things are even more complex. Individual agents and clients find themselves acting in ways constrained by the way those around them do things. But their responses to how things are done will differ. For instance, if managers restrict physicians' treatment options according to the cost of some procedures, say, physicians in two different hospitals or two different wards will do things in different ways, even though complying with the same directive. However, each of them will form somewhat different attitudes to the need to avoid using the proscribed procedures. These differing attitudes colour how they do things. For instance, one physician may comply with a directive in a grudging and complaining manner, while another physician is more accepting and given to exploring alternatives. These differences will feed back on how things are done in the particular ward or hospital, in that one or another attitude may be taken up by others and become dominant, defining the work environment of the hospital or ward.

Physicians working in a hospital located in an economically depressed community may comply with restrictive directives but attempt to circumvent them when they can, because they feel that their patients' lot is already bad enough and should not be worsened by what they see as bureaucratic miserliness. Physicians working in a hospital located in an affluent community may disagree with the restrictive directives, but nonetheless comply with them and not attempt to circumvent them. Again, physicians dealing mainly with women or mainly with men will deal with the directives somewhat differently, as is the case where race or economic class is a dominant factor. But all of this has to do with what the physicians do in direct response to the directives; there is more that goes on. The directives may dishearten the physicians working in the economically depressed community. They may begin to feel that the practice of medicine is being jeopardized by what they see as bureaucratic waste and lack of understanding, and this perception will affect how they do things. The physicians in the affluent community, buoyed up by the generally good health of their patients – due in significant part to better nutrition and level of education – may see the directives as reasonable measures. Gender-specific situations further complicate things. A case in point is the standard test for prostate cancer. In Ontario, the test is not covered by provincial insurance, unless prescribed by the physician, and is offered as an option that costs about twenty dollars. This is a notable instance because virtually all cancer-screening procedures for women are covered. Physicians in the depressed community may deplore having their male patients, many of whom are unemployed, pay for a test they think prudent, if not necessary. They then may find ways of justifying the prescribing of the test in order to save their patients the cost. On the other hand, physicians in the affluent community may think nothing of the cost to their patients and simply recommend the test. Age may enter the picture, too, in that physicians in either community may forgo ordering some screening tests for women of advanced age because, even though covered, they are expensive.

The case of patients is somewhat simpler because their options are more limited. Nonetheless, they do things in ways partly determined by how and what health care managers and practitioners do. Consider again the case of tests done at patients' expense. Patients in the affluent community, for whom the amounts are relatively trivial, may not only not hesitate to have the tests done, but do so eagerly, thinking that they are doing something proactive regarding their health. Patients in the economically depressed community may have no option but to forgo the tests because they cannot pay for them or because they resent having to pay for what they see as part of care to which they are entitled, or to go to some effort to find the money. Each of these choices has repercussions for individuals' health and the health of the community. And there is another sort of consequence. Having the tests done, and paying for them, may make patients in the affluent community see themselves as fortunate to be able to take a hand in maintaining their health. The patients in the economically depressed community may feel demeaned by being put in a situation where they must either forgo something that is in their interests or go to considerable effort to achieve it. These different attitudinal responses are cumulative. That is, after a time they come to define individuals' self-images and so the character of a community.

Three elements or factors in the foregoing – what managers do, what practitioners and patients do, and the attitudes all of these individuals adopt in doing what they do – combine in what basically are unpredictable ways. As a result, health care is affected in various ways. Consider just one example. Imagine that physicians working in the economically depressed community regularly circumvent the restrictive directive regarding the prostate cancer screening test. Though the test was judged to be normally unnecessary and classified as elective, many of the physicians strongly disagree with that assessment. Imagine further that the physicians, resentful of how they are being made to practise in an economically depressed community, knowingly or unknowingly justify prescribing the test by overestimating risks and overemphasizing their diagnostic suspicions. The initial assessment of the test as unnecessary in most cases was based on statistical data. The physicians' circumvention of the directive, then, results in their practice being out of line with the projections operant in implementation of the directive. One result is that the expected savings are not realized. But another result is that due to the expected savings not being realized, managers commission a new statistical study to establish what went amiss. Physicians' extensive prescription of the test now skews the figures regarding the apparent necessity of a test judged normally unnecessary on the basis of earlier figures. A new directive is issued and patients no longer need pay for the test. The result is that a test that likely is in fact normally not necessary comes to be used more extensively, which drives costs up. Ultimately, a cost-cutting measure ends up raising costs.

Below we will pursue one aspect of the foregoing, which is that regardless of their assigned roles and status, agents and clients redefine themselves relative to how health care affects each of them and, as important, how they *perceive* it affects them. As a consequence, inevitable differences develop between, on the one hand, the agents and clients the planners had in mind, and that managers think they are dealing with, and, on the other hand, the actual agents and clients. Above we alluded to this by saying that some agents may grow resentful of how they must work, and some clients may feel demeaned by being put in certain positions. The point is that each agent and client has a unique history that conditions how he or she responds to imposed control. This is as important as the fact that each is affected by others' behaviour. But in addition to having a unique history – a history that encompasses rearing, education, gender, race, religious commitment, political orientation, and so on – each agent or client is engaged, to a greater or lesser extent, in a process of self-definition. Their responses to feeling resentful or demeaned, then, will vary with how their histories and those efforts at self-definition mesh with one another.

To continue with our more abstract presentation, Foucault's genealogical work focuses on how institutions mould their agents and clients in the process of classifying, regulating, and controlling them. To say how this works Foucault wrote *Discipline and Punish* and the first volume of *The History of Sexuality*. We must characterize the process much more briefly.

The basic idea is an ancient one: imposing behavioural habits on individuals not only controls their behaviour, it shapes or reshapes their perspectives, attitudes, values, desires, and other affective aspects. Foucault adds the realization that imposition of behavioural habits is most effective in institutional contexts: the prison, the convent, the school, the barracks, the hospital, the factory.[9] In these, especially in the prison, there developed "what might be called the political technology of the body."[10] For Foucault, the point of the technology is not just control, which is achievable through restrictions and prohibitions; the point is pervasive management. What is new in Foucault's consideration of management is description of how it is achieved both with restrictions and with enabling conceptions, definitions, and descriptions that support behaviour-governing norms. What is also new is description of modern management as needing the complicity of those managed. Complicity is needed because what is sought is not just obedience, but deep internalization of a carefully designed understanding of the self. Foucault describes five devices used to achieve this end:

- Hierarchical observation
- Normalizing judgment
- The examination
- Panopticism
- Surveillance

Of these, the device that best captures the process of imposing habits on people is panopticism; it is the one we will discuss in greatest detail. The others can be more briefly described.

Hierarchical observation involves physically structuring spaces to maximize the ability of those in authority to oversee what goes on in a particular environment. An example is a work area with elevated positions for supervisors. In *Discipline and Punish*, Foucault considers several examples, like tiered lecture halls, but contemporary audio-visual devices have superseded most of them. The core of hierarchical observation is the enabling of individuals of higher rank in an institution to easily observe the activities of individuals of lower rank.

Normalizing judgment is comparative negative assessment of individuals or groups. Though not outright criticism or condemnation, it is invidious comparison with a favoured individual or group. A case in point is glorifying a particular team as a model of high productivity, and then simply letting it stand as an example to be emulated by any other team. Nothing specific need be said about the exemplary team's makeup or how it functions; it suffices that it is extolled in various ways. Specific comparisons can remain tacit, as everyone will draw them. It merits mention that this is one area where failure to consider the role of gender poses a particularly serious shortfall.

The examination is use of all kinds of tests the results of which enable tighter classification and control. An example is placement tests that categorize new students, employees, or inmates, and justify their being assigned to certain groups, given certain duties, and treated in certain ways. As important is that test results define individuals in various ways and influence their choices and expectations.

Surveillance, of course, is all sorts of direct and electronic observation by those in authority and by peers. However, Foucault extends surveillance to the keeping of files on people, to predicting their behaviour on the basis of tests, and to enabling acceptance of the idea that there are experts who know more about individuals than they know about themselves.

Panopticism derives from Jeremy Bentham's design for an ideal prison, the Panopticon, which embodies the idea that "the fact of being constantly seen, of being able always to be seen ... maintains the disciplined individual in his subjugation."[11] In Bentham's prison, cells are arranged around a central observation tower. Inmates are always observable to watchers in the tower, but the inmates cannot see their observers. The practical effect is the same as continuous surveillance. The inmates are constantly vulnerable to vigilance and its sanctions, so they must behave as if constantly observed. But Foucault expands on Bentham's idea, contending that surveillance can turn unwilling submission to directives into willing conformity with norms. This idea has two parts. The first is that panopticism can convert deliberate obedience of regulations into habitual compliance with norms. The second part is that habitual compliance itself converts to adoption or "internalization" of the norms in question.

Because the term "panopticism" is so closely tied to penal institutions, despite Foucault's generalization of the notion, we will speak of *monitoring* in what follows. Perhaps the simplest and most familiar example of monitoring, of how "being able always to be seen" keeps disciplined individuals subjugated and instills habits in them, is Santa Claus. As the Christmas carol "Santa Claus Is Coming to Town" tells children, Santa sees them when they are sleeping and knows when they are awake, so the carol urges them "to be good, for goodness' sake." Santa is always monitoring their behaviour, so they must behave as if always observed. The Santa Claus story has all the central Foucauldian elements. It is presented to children as a charming tale and an enhancement to holiday cheer, but it actually serves to impose control on their behaviour. Children cannot always be watched, so various devices are used that get them to remain compliant to behavioural directives while they are not being watched. But the story does not only impose compliance. Its presentation is value-laden, and the child complies, not simply with specific directives, but with the model of the well-behaved youngster who is rewarded for being good. In complying with directives and monitoring themselves, children are formed, and form themselves, as "good" children. They come to aspire to being the model of the well-behaved youngster and, to a greater or lesser extent, they become the model.

A simple example in health care has to do with how patients are deluged with dietary information designed to alter their eating habits. As we see around us every day, marketers have been quick to capitalize on this, and they have succeeded so well that we do not find it absurd when a fruit-juice label trumpets the fact that the juice contains no cholesterol. People eating ice cream find it necessary either to joke about what they are doing or to assure themselves that they have earned the forbidden treat. Individuals having little idea of what a protein is nonetheless talk about high-density lipoproteins to justify drinking an extra glass of wine. Monitoring is evident in these cases. Whether or not the individuals are complying with dietary directives, they are monitoring themselves. Not eating ice cream because of worries about cholesterol, having an ice cream and justifying it, or just having it and feeling guilty are all the same with respect to monitoring. In all three cases, what individuals actually do is done in a context established by admonitions against saturated fats. Few people who have been warned by their doctors to reduce their cholesterol levels are able to have a bacon-and-eggs breakfast without thinking much about it. In this they reveal themselves to be complicitous in their own monitoring; they are "inmates" of a controlling institution and colluding in medical and nutritional surveillance of themselves. We could go on for many pages giving examples of how health care managers or physicians monitor themselves in light of institutional directives, professional standards, peer expectations, and patient demands. Below we consider a case in point of how monitoring works and has significant consequences. The point, though, should be clear. Monitoring is how an institution changes and forms its agents and clients by getting them to watch themselves for compliance with its principles and regulations.

However, monitoring does not occur in a vacuum. However structured and regulated by institutions, human interactions are very complex, and Foucault also is concerned to describe how human interactions have random or "accidental" consequences. The import of this is that those consequences condition how monitoring works and how effective it is. Foucault has a good deal to say about how what individuals do is unintentionally and incidentally affected by what others do. Discipline always is imposed in contexts of mostly unwitting and unrecognized mutual influencing of one another by those who impose discipline and those who are disciplined. The point here is that all the while that institutions are trying to shape individuals into compliant subjects, those individuals are being variously influenced by others' actions. This convoluted interaction is what genealogy traces and is what Foucault calls power relations or power. But things are further complicated by the fact that while individuals are being shaped by institutional discipline, and being influenced by others' actions, they are deliberately trying to shape themselves into subjects of their choosing. These latter endeavours are what Foucault considers in his ethics.

We have identified three major elements or features of health care's dynamics:

- Institutional shaping of agents' and clients' subjectivity
- Mutual influencing among agents and clients
- Agents' and clients' efforts at self-determination

We will expand on these; what we need to do now is say how these elements jointly determine the very nature of health care as an enterprise. In other words, we have to discuss power or power relations, and we do so in the next chapter.

CHAPTER TWO

Health Care and Power

In *Madness and Civilization* Foucault considers institutionalized exclusionary, manipulative, and restrictive treatment of the insane. In *The Birth of the Clinic* he considers institutionalized exclusionary, manipulative, and therapeutic treatment of the physically afflicted. In *Discipline and Punish* he considers institutionalized exclusionary, manipulative, and rehabilitative treatment of lawbreakers. In *The History of Sexuality*, volume 1, he considers the socially constructed nature of sexuality. The deeper focus of these works, especially *Discipline and Punish*, is how disciplinary techniques develop and work to control populations segregated either physically or through classification and categorization, and how those techniques redefine the members of those populations.

Circumscription of a group through classification is the initial step in the management, or what Foucault calls the "government," of subjects.[1] As noted in the previous chapter, subjects are individuals who are *subjective* entities in being self-aware individuals, and who also are *subjected* entities in being individuals subordinate to society and the state. Subjects are identified as members of a designated population: the sick, the mad, the criminal. What Foucault offers that is new is that he sees this identification or classification not as discernment of existing conditions, but as the social construction of abnormalities.[2] He describes classification as knitting together of particular behavioural traits into claimed manifestations of deviancy from the norms of health, sanity, and social responsibility. However, we need not pursue the controversial constructivist side of Foucault's work. What is important here is classification itself, whatever its grounds. The crucial point is that once classification occurs, it enables the second step in management or government of groups or designated populations, which is institutional isolation of individuals in hospitals, asylums, penitentiaries, and similar establishments. Isolation, though, does not have to be achieved by quartering people in so many buildings; it can be achieved symbolically by the application of designations and categories. As is shown in the first volume of *The History of Sexuality*, a group need not be physically sequestered to be circumscribed. Individuals can be grouped and marked as a designated population within the general population through application of labels denoting aberrations. For instance, classification and symbolic isolation of individuals who engage in homosexual activity as deviants not only establishes an aberrant nature, it automatically establishes heterosexuality as "natural" and the norm. Symbolic isolation applies even where individuals are physically sequestered in one or another institution; types of treatment, prognoses, duties, privileges, and sentences further delineate groups among the inmates of hospitals, asylums, or prisons.

Once a group has been circumscribed and physically and/or symbolically isolated, the third step in designated-population management is imposition of discipline. In the case of the sick and insane, discipline is integral to treatment and avowedly therapeutic; in the case of the criminal, discipline is integral to preventive and punitive confinement and avowedly rehabilatory. In all cases, discipline is imposed directly, by directive, and indirectly, by the establishment of norms and normalizing devices such as counselling. Discipline's avowed purpose is to benefit the members of the target groups, whether through therapy or rehabilitation. Contrary to this, Foucault claims that discipline's real purpose is control through normalization. In this connection, he stresses two points. First, control is not achieved just through imposition of proscriptions and restrictions; it is also achieved through enabling descriptions and self-images. That is, effective control does not only prohibit, it facilitates and encourages select ways of behaving and preferred ways of thinking of oneself. Second, effective control requires the complicity of those controlled if it is to be prescriptive as well as proscriptive. Individuals being controlled must not merely conform to regulations and imposed practices because they fear the consequences of not doing so. They must want to conform; they must see conforming as the right thing to do. They must adopt and internalize the prescriptive elements, the enabling descriptions and self-images. For instance, prison inmates must not only behave as prison authorities require, they must come to see themselves as having acted sociopathologically, as deserving incarceration and needing rehabilitation for their own sake as well as for others' good. Complicity is achieved when disciplined subjects internalize a carefully constructed value-laden understanding of themselves as having a certain nature, and as needing to conform to that nature and to rectify having deviated from it. Adoption of the fostered self-conception then determines subjects' behaviour by making them want to be normal, by making them want to act in conformity with their nature and to avoid deviancy.

Both those who impose discipline and those who are disciplined exist in a complex environment generated by the actions of others as well as their own actions. It is with regard to this complex mutual influencing that Foucault's concept of power or power relations enables us to better comprehend how subjects are shaped not only by discipline but also by interaction with others. Unfortunately, Foucault's concept of power is elusive. This is in part because of the concept's novelty and difficulty, and in part because of a strong tendency on most people's part to understand Foucauldian power as we ordinarily understand power, that is, as the state's or a group's or an individual's capability to coerce and command. More specifically, Foucauldian power often is misunderstood as covert domination of people in institutional contexts. But Foucauldian power is not the capability to make anyone do anything; it is not force nor capacity nor domination nor authority. Foucault insists on "the strictly relational character of power relationships."[3] He insists further that "power is not ... a certain strength."[4] Instead of Foucauldian power being coercive or commanding or intimidating force, it is a "set of actions upon other actions."[5] Power or power relations are not persuasion or coercion exercised by individuals or groups on other individuals or groups. Most simply put, power is people doing things and what they do affecting others and what those others do. As we explain below, to grasp the concept of Foucauldian power, one needs to refocus from people doing things to the things people do. We normally focus primarily on individuals acting in various ways; Foucault requires that we bring the acts themselves into the foreground and push the individuals who act into the background.

Once we focus on acts, rather than on those who act, we begin to understand how power is "actions upon other actions." Focusing on actions enables us to grasp a point that is essential to Foucault's conception of power. The point is that contrary to our usual way of thinking about power, Foucauldian power is not exercised by anyone because it is not *exercised* at all. It is not something that is applied or exerted; rather, it is dynamic, continuous change in networks of inter-related actions. This is how Foucauldian power "is a way in which certain actions modify other [actions]," and why power "does not act directly and immediately on others," acting instead "upon their actions."[6] Cases of the application of power in the ordinary sense, as when one person coerces another to do something or an institution requires its inmates to comply with a schedule, are only components of the latticework that is Foucauldian power. These components are the actions that affect other actions. An important consequence is that unlike ordinary power, which is someone's or some group's ability to achieve certain ends, Foucauldian power is impersonal and blind. That is, power serves no one's ends because power is no one's power. Power has no objectives, and it has direction only in the sense that the effects of its component actions are cumulative over time.

Though difficult, it is crucial to grasp Foucault's conception of power as impersonal and hence not a capacity or force that is brought to bear on individuals or groups. It needs to be understood that in Foucauldian power relations, actions are constrained by other actions at a level different from that at which one or more individuals control what others do. Foucauldian power must be understood as "imma-nent in force relationships" rather than as itself a compelling force possessed and exerted by an individual or a group or the state.[7] This point is particularly important to grasp in order to understand how interactions in health care have consequences that no one anticipated or intended to bring about. The idea that the actual outcome of a policy or directive is either what someone in authority intended, or the result of error or obstruction, is too simple. Many of the conse-quences of implemented policies and directives are what they are because of how people interact with one another, because of how their actions bear on the actions of others.

The point here is that the importance of power's impersonal nature is that since it is no one's power, the effects of institutional disciplines on designated populations ultimately are and can be only partially intentional. Once grasped, this basic Foucauldian point explains how health care's management may go wrong even though flawlessly applied. The problem is that managers operate in an environment of power relations, so not only are their actions constrained by others' actions, their actions bear on individuals who are influenced by the actions of those around them. That is, the actions that constitute the managing of an enterprise occur in a complex network of other actions, and those other actions constrain both the managing actions and the actions that are individuals' responses to the managing. This means that those who are managed will not be motivated and regulated precisely as managers intend them to be. Moreover, this genealogical point has to be complemented with an ethical one, in Foucault's sense of "ethical." Though a discussion of Foucauldian ethics is still to come, it must be kept in mind that people respond to being managed in ways determined in part by their own unique life histories, gender, age, and economic circumstances, and in part by their own efforts to be certain sorts of persons.

The impersonality of power, or what Foucault calls its "non-subjective" character, is not really as peculiar as it initially appears.[8] When we think of people engaged in an activity, we naturally focus on them doing various things. But as noted above, to understand Foucauldian power we need to focus on the actions themselves, instead of on individuals doing what they are doing. We have to look past the individuals, the agents, to see the dynamic and fluid lacework of interrelated acts that those individuals generate in acting as they do. Foucauldian power is the lacework. When we see it as such, we understand how power relations or power is "a total structure of actions brought to bear upon possible actions."[9] What this means is that power, the total structure of actions, enables or facilitates some actions and inhibits or precludes others.[10] This also clarifies Foucault's use of the term "constraint." The term usually means restriction or limitation, but, like "power," Foucault uses the term in a more abstract or extensive way. Actions are constrained in that, as just said, some are enabled or facilitated while others are inhibited or precluded. That is, one individual's actions make it more or less likely that another individual will or will not do something, or will or will not do something in a certain way. Foucault makes the single term "constrain" work as do pairs of terms like facilitate/impede, encourage/inhibit, and permit/hinder.

A simple example will prove helpful. Imagine sitting in a crowded theatre. If the person on your left is leaning too close to you, you can ask that person to move a little. Doing that would be to act on him or her by making a request and, assuming compliance, making him or her do something. Our sense of personal space is strong, but our responses to most incursions are largely unconscious; for instance, we usually respond to slight crowding more or less unthinkingly. What is most likely is that you will lean away from your closely seated seatmate without thinking about it. But then you unwittingly invade the personal space of the person seated on your right. That person likely will lean away from you, also without thinking, and so unintentionally invade the next person's space. Eventually, everyone in the row will be leaning to the right, and probably with little awareness of doing so. Your left-hand neighbour's action of leaning to the right resulted in you leaning to the right, and your action in turn resulted in your right-hand seatmate leaning to the right. There were other options, like complaining or changing seats, but the action of leaning to the right is the one made most likely by the initial action and the context in which it occurred. Put in Foucauldian terms, your actions were constrained by your left-hand neighbour's action in that your leaning to the right was made very likely, whereas your leaning to the left was made very unlikely. The result is that everyone in the row ends up leaning to the right, not at your left-hand seatmate's request or command, but in response to his or her action of leaning to the right. This is the sense in which power is actions acting on actions.

An example in the health care area, alluded to above, needs to be a bit more complicated. For one thing, as noted earlier, factors such as gender and age are always operant. For another, practices not only vary a good deal from hospital to hospital, clinic to clinic, and even from ward to ward, they are constantly changing. Consider that nurses now routinely carry stethoscopes, as various tasks that once were the exclusive prerogative of physicians have been delegated to nurses with the appropriate training. However, not long ago, wearing a stethoscope was a badge of office exclusive to physicians and interns. Imagine the following situation arising at a time when wearing a stethoscope was something that only physicians and interns were privileged to do. A hospital hires a consultant to deal with its nursing staff's low morale. One of the issues that emerge is that the nurses think the hospital's physicians too aloof and even arrogant. The consultant runs some sensitivity-heightening sessions for the physicians, and one of the examples used in the sessions is that of the doctors wearing their stethoscopes on rounds. The consultant's point is that doing so is perceived by the nurses as flaunting their status. Some months later, a young female doctor joins the staff. The new doctor is accustomed to wearing her stethoscope on rounds, as did a doctor she knew in her residency, whom she considers her mentor, and whom she tries to emulate. However, unless actually using them, her new colleagues pocket their stethoscopes while on rounds. This is done as a result of the consultant's efforts, but the new doctor is not told that because no one thinks to do so. However, the new doctor, like the theatre-goer, unthinkingly begins to pocket her stethoscope on rounds. After a few days she notices that several nurses who had been aloof earlier now treat her in a friendlier manner. She puts this down to the nurses becoming more familiar with her, since she knows nothing about the consultant. She is also unaware that not only is wearing a stethoscope on rounds irksome to some nurses and others, but that doing so acquired special significance because of being used by the consultant as an example of workplace insensitivity. Several months later, a renowned surgeon is wooed away from a prestigious clinic and joins the staff. The surgeon wears his stethoscope on rounds, as he has always done, and pays no attention to how his new colleagues pocket theirs. Soon some of the other doctors begin wearing their stethoscopes on rounds, as they did before the consultant was hired. Eventually the hospital's physicians are again wearing their stethoscopes on rounds. Some do so without thinking; some genuinely find it more convenient; some resent having had to change what seems to them an innocuous habit. The young doctor also slips back into her earlier habit of wearing her stethoscope on rounds. The nurses, having had their expectations raised by the consultant's efforts, not only see renewal of the practice as reassertion of attitudes they deplore, they see the young doctor's wearing of her stethoscope as a special case of a woman doctor showing insensitivity or indifference to their concerns. The wearing of stethoscopes, a very minor matter in its own right, assumes a disproportionate importance and becomes a magnifying lens through which other practices and events are perceived as much more insensitive than they are. The upshot is that the nurses' morale drops even lower than prior to the consultant's being hired.

What is important here is that in some cases we do what we do, not because we are told or forced to do it, but because of changes in the situation we find ourselves in. Foucault's way of putting this point is to say that sometimes we do what we do, not because we are told or forced to do it, but because the power relations we find ourselves in are altered by someone's actions. In this sense, power is the sum total of influences that actions, not agents, have on other actions. Power, as "a total structure of actions brought to bear upon possible actions," is actions affecting other actions by enabling or encouraging some behaviour and inhibiting or discouraging other behaviour.[11] An action may be enabled or encouraged, as when someone senior takes off a jacket at a meeting in an overly warm room and, by doing so, makes it possible for you to remove yours. An action may be inhibited or discouraged, as when your lunch guest orders club soda and you do not order the glass of wine you intended to order. In the theatre case, one theatre-goer leaning to the right does not force the right-hand neighbour to also lean right. The first person's leaning to the right is an action that makes the second theatre-goer's leaning to the right the likeliest response among a set of possible actions, which include possible but more immoderate options like complaining or changing seats.

The stethoscope example illustrates power relations as does the theatre case, but it also shows how one individual's efforts at self-determination complicate matters. The young female doctor tries to be like the physician she admires. Wearing her stethoscope on rounds is a small action that fits better with her efforts to do so than does pocketing her stethoscope. Therefore, though she initially pocketed her stethoscope in line with what her new colleagues did, she is quick to wear it on rounds when other doctors begin do so.

Once the idea of power as the network of actions bearing on actions is grasped, it becomes evident why Foucault maintains that power relations "permeate ... and constitute the social body."[12] We are social creatures, and we have our being as social creatures in an environment of power relations; everything we do is influenced by what others do. None of us is ever free of power relations because none of us is ever truly alone in the sense of being outside a social structure. Even when we are alone, we are bound by our enculturation as social beings. Alone on his island, Robinson Crusoe could go about naked and leave his possessions anywhere he wanted. Crusoe was temporarily free of power relations because there was no one else on the island whose actions constrained his actions. But Crusoe was still a social being. When he saw a footprint on the beach, he suddenly dressed and stored his possessions. The footprint activated a network of potential power relations, even though he had not actually seen anyone. The mere sign of another person's possible presence sufficed to constrain Crusoe's actions, because it sufficed to re-establish his compliance with social norms. Even though fictional, the Crusoe case illustrates the monitoring so central to Foucault's thinking. Crusoe's behaviour illustrates how individuals who internalize norms monitor themselves for compliance. No one forced Crusoe to put on clothes or put away his few things. He did so because that is what one does in the company of others. Crusoe behaved *normally*, and he was complicit in his own social control. He wanted to conform because he saw doing so as the right thing to do, and saw not doing so as deviant.

What Foucault describes as normalization is most evident in *The History of Sexuality*, where he traces the establishment of heterosexual procreative activity as the essence of sexual normalcy, and the designation of other sexual activity as deviant. In *Discipline and Punish*, as discussed above, Foucault considers normalization in terms of the inspired realization that surveillance by others can be turned into self-surveillance. The key to doing so is establishing the illusion of "being always to be seen." Subjects are made complicit in their own monitoring by being made to believe themselves always under observation. Subjects' complicity in their own control then is increased by imposing on them the "obligation to seek and state the truth about oneself."[13] This is part of "the examination," and involves interviews, questionnaires, and counselling sessions that are presented as diagnostic and therapeutic devices, but really serve to instill in subjects a certain picture of who they are and who they should be. This is how "discipline produces ... 'docile' bodies."[14] Additionally, by imposing behaviour that is presented as being in conformity with nature, discipline identifies and stigmatizes deviant behaviour.[15]

However, while normalization is tremendously effective, it also introduces a measure of unpredictability. This is because the norms an institution or society tries to inculcate in subjects may be altered or distorted by how individuals actually internalize them. One decisive factor is how power relations have previously shaped individuals, and so determined how those individuals construe and adapt the norms they internalize.

We can summarize the foregoing points as follows: managing designated populations – the sick, the insane, the criminal – involves exclusionary classification, physical or symbolic segregation, and disciplinary techniques designed to achieve normalization. Some people are set apart by being classed together and/or institutionalized to better control them and to contain whatever makes them problematic: the disruptive inconsistency of the insane, the disconcerting dependence of the sick, the menacing sociopathology of the criminal. The objective is to normalize the selected individuals, to render them unproblematic by restraining, curing, or rehabilitating them. Doing so is achieved by imposing discipline that complements treatment, structures their activities, and shapes and controls their behaviour. Normalizing discipline culminates in making individuals monitor their own conformity to the norms the discipline inculcates.

It must be kept in mind, though, that normalization rarely is a knowingly undertaken, deliberately striven for objective. Its attempted attainment appears to those who impose normalizing discipline as a matter of curing, rehabilitating, improving, and even liberating individuals in designated populations. Normalization itself simply is the sum of the disciplinary actions taken by those in authority over members of a segregated population and the influence of actions by peers. At the institutional level, normalization is the sum of instances of imposing schedules, examining and diagnosing patients, prescribing activities or medication, counselling inmates, administering tests, and so on. At the policy level, normalization is the sum of assessments and evaluations of situations, the determination of ends, the structuring of a service or remedial program, and the devising of disciplines to achieve objectives. There is no conspiracy to normalize patients or inmates; there are just efforts – quite genuine efforts – *to make things better*, and those efforts all involve disciplining individuals who are judged to be in some way abnormal.

Normalizing discipline proceeds primarily through application of the devices Foucault lists: hierarchical observation, normalizing judgment, the examination, panopticism – which we are calling *monitoring* – and surveillance. However, normalizing discipline has two problematic dimensions of special interest to us. First, it is conducted in an environment of power relations, so disciplinary actions are constrained by other actions, and those actions may be done in ways that fail to achieve their intended ends. Second, the individuals who are disciplined each have their own unique histories and are in the process of trying to be the persons they want to be. Therefore, a significant measure of disruptive unpredictability is generated by how individuals respond to normalizing discipline imposed by their physicians, psychiatrists, wardens, and anyone else involved in their supervision.

The way the foregoing bears on health care is that health care management is not merely a matter of administering services, marshalling and allocating resources, and delivering various forms of treatment. Health care management is Foucauldian government of a large number of people and involves normalization. Health care's agents and clients are members of tightly interrelated designated populations. Agents are categorized in numerous ways: as directors, administrators, surgeons, general practitioners, registered nurses, nurses' aides, paramedics, and so on. They are assigned credentials attesting to various sorts and levels of expertise. They are spatially circumscribed as health care providers in that they perform their duties in hospitals, clinics, health centres, sanatoriums, infirmaries, nursing homes, and doctors' offices. They must meet both institutional and professional standards; they must conform to the cultures of individual hospitals, clinics, wards, and even medical office buildings; the procedures they perform are precisely delineated; their conduct must accord with peers' practices. Each hospital, clinic, and ward imposes discipline on its operatives, scheduling their time, prescribing their duties, and imposing on them corporate objectives. Moreover, beyond all of the explicit managing directives are the implicit ones that defy enumeration. These are all the expectations and subtle demands arising from entrenched attitudes regarding such factors as gender.

On the client side, patients are categorized according to their afflictions, age, gender, insurance status, and so on, and are further classified as in-patients, out-patients, chronic cases, acute cases, terminal cases, ambulatory, bedridden, and the like. Most notably, patients are virtually identified with their charts, and their charts include information with definite normative implications, such as do-not-resuscitate orders and whether they are compliant or not compliant. Patients are spatially circumscribed, in that they are interviewed, examined, counselled, and treated in hospitals, clinics, and doctors' offices, and, if hospitalized, are assigned to particular wards. Patients are expected to comply willingly with instructions and admonitions about medication dosages, diet, exercise, personal hygiene, and psychological attitudes. Compliance involves not only following instructions, but also the implicit expectations and demands, many of them gender- and age-related, such as being quiet, maintaining a measure of cheerfulness, not being demanding, not questioning treatment decisions, and not being "difficult" with respect to providing informed consent for procedures.

Health care management, then, involves normalization and discipline. But like all other activities, health care management operates in a context of power relations. Moreover, it deals with agents and clients each of whom has been somewhat differently shaped by power relations, is somewhat differently affected by others' actions, and is engaged in self-determination to one or another extent. All of this means that health care management does not go wrong only for extrinsic reasons such as people inevitably making mistakes, having limited knowledge, acting self-interestedly, and innocently or deliberately thwarting others' efforts. Health care management also goes wrong because it is conducted in an environment of power relations, and because its agents and clients each respond a little differently to being managed. How things go wrong in these second and third ways has little to do with errors, ignorance, opportunism, or obstructiveness. Instead, how things go wrong in these two ways has everything to do with Foucauldian power and Foucauldian ethics.

We can articulate much that we already understand about health care – even if only inchoately – in Foucauldian terms in the following way. Health care is managed in an environment of previous and contemporaneous constraining actions; that is, health care is managed in a latticework of power relations. This is to say that past and present actions condition, shape, and direct the actions that specifically constitute the managing of health care at any given time. In addition, the individuals who are managed, that is, health care's agents and clients, respond to being managed in light of how they are influenced by others' actions. Moreover, how they respond is further affected by how they perceive themselves acting and how they feel they should act. The consequence of these several influences is that neither managers nor anyone else can adequately map the latticework of power relations that they modify and contribute to in acting as they do. The results of their efforts, then, are essentially unpredictable. We pursue the nature of this unpredictability in the next chapter, but it can be clarified here with another example.

Administrators need to increase a small hospital's efficiency in light of a provincial cost-cutting plan to close hospitals that are judged redundant. Among other things, they impose a schedule on staff physicians, limiting the time they may spend with individual patients on rounds. The schedule is worked out on the basis of national and provincial statistics on time physicians normally spend with various sorts of patients, correlated with the hospital's own records. However, staff physicians have previously given generously of their time, arriving at the hospital earlier and leaving later than required or reported. The reason is that the hospital is in an economically depressed area and the physicians feel a heightened obligation to their patients. Additionally, a highly respected and dedicated member of the staff sets a daunting example for colleagues. The hospital's physicians, therefore, see more patients than they otherwise would see, despite seeing patients for longer periods than the statistical averages. Both the number of patients seen and the time spent with each are important because the average level of education in the community is low, and many of the patients need basic health care information – especially about birth control and safe sex – beyond the specific treatments they receive. The physicians, conscious of the need, take every opportunity to instruct the patients they see, to prescribe birth control pills, and even to dispense condoms.

When the new schedule is imposed, the hospital's physicians resent it because they see it as an intrusion on their practice of medicine and because of how they have been generous with their time. But they do not oppose the schedule in any organized way, seeing it as evidence of administrative insensitivity and thinking opposition to be pointless. Instead they adhere to the schedule and stop working extended hours, thus seeing fewer patients and seeing each for less time than before. The outcome is that instead of bringing about an increase in efficiency, in terms of the number of patients seen, the schedule actually decreases efficiency. The schedule also introduces unproductive tensions between the administration and the physicians. Most importantly, the hospital's contribution to the well-being of its community decreases, narrowing considerably to the provision of reactive care. As an indirect consequence of the hospital's narrower contribution to the community, there are small but significant and noted increases in teenage pregnancies and HIV cases in the community. The hospital's drop in efficiency, and the worsening local health statistics, eventually result in the province moving to close the hospital and expanding the services of a nearby larger one. And because members of the community perceive a new indifference to their needs on the part of the hospital's physicians, electoral support for keeping the hospital open proves inadequate. In this way, the imposition of a schedule intended to help prevent the hospital's being closed in fact contributes significantly to it being closed.

In this example, the physicians' working unreported hours represents actions that constrain the administrators' action of imposing the schedule. The physicians' actions represent the power relations in which the administrators act. The fact that the physicians' extra work is not reported represents how planning and implementation of policy often misses or misconstrues one or another local condition that impedes or precludes success. The physicians' resentment of the schedule represents the way in which individuals' perceptions, preferences, and proclivities determine how they respond to being managed. The example as a whole represents how an action done with a specific objective in mind may have unpredictable consequences because of the context in which it is done.

AN INTERIM SUMMARY

It may be useful here to reiterate that, given the difficulty and elusiveness of Foucault's thought, and especially of his concept of power, repetition is necessary in exposition because we need to come at the same points from several slightly different angles in order to make them as accessible as possible.

As suggested, there is a sense in which we have always known much of what Foucault articulates about human interaction and behaviour. What happens in any complex human interaction is a vector product; that is, what happens has multiple causes. What happens has as many causes as there are individuals whose actions bear on what happens. Moreover, some causes enhance other active causes, while some causes inhibit or nullify still others, thereby increasing the causal complexity. And only some, perhaps very few, of the contributing causes are evident or traceable. Not everything that bears on what happens can be identified as just this or that action by a particular individual, and what individuals do strengthens or weakens the effect of what others do in ways we cannot begin to track.

But event sequences are even more complex, because the multiple causes of individuals' actions are themselves vector products; that is, each contributing action is itself a complex effect of three different sorts of causes. First, individuals are made or required to do certain things by employers, friends, relatives, agents of various institutions and the state, and – of greatest relevance here – those caring for them. Second, individuals are influenced to do certain things, and to do them in certain ways, by the impact on them of what others do. Third, individuals are led to assume particular roles and choose specific courses of action by their own histories, perceptions, fears, and aspirations.

Foucault's notion of power or power relations is a device to enable better understanding of behavioural vector products, of how complex human interactions produce the results they do, and of how individuals do the things they do. The notion of power is the core of genealogical analysis, and it functions to trace how institutions work and produce the results they produce, especially with respect to how they affect and shape their people. It is in these analyses that Foucault exposes what Rorty describes as constraints not dreamt of by premodern societies.[16] Foucault's ethical contentions – in his self-oriented sense of "ethical" – are about how individuals strive to make themselves into subjects all the while that they are being shaped by various institutions and disciplines. The importance for us of the ethical contentions is that individuals' efforts at self-determination play a significant contributing role in how they behave in institutional settings, in general, and how they behave as providers and recipients of health care, in particular.

Foucault's contentions about power relations and self-determination, especially the former, are made in the context of his historical observation that at some time within the last two or three centuries, we made ourselves objects of study. We began to develop human science; we not only objectified ourselves, we began to seek law-like generalizations about our behaviour. We began to learn a great deal about ourselves – Foucault would say to *construct* a great deal about ourselves – and so about controlling people with techniques going far beyond threats and shows of force. The new control turns on inculcating certain conceptions and perceptions of self in those to be controlled. The first step in exercising the new control is designation or selection. That is, individuals need to be grouped on the basis of whatever representatives of the majority think makes them problematic, and whatever that may be, it is interpreted as deviancy, hence the introduction of classifications or categories: the criminal, the infirm, the irrational. Ideally, for maximum control, those grouped by being identified as somehow deviant are physically separated from the general population in prisons, hospitals, asylums, and similar institutions. But the disciplinary techniques work so well in institutional contexts that they inevitably are extended beyond confining walls to institutions in a broader sense, namely, education, the military, the business world, the political sphere. Extending discipline in this way requires symbolic designation and classification. If it is unworkable to separate out people by physically confining them, they must be separated out through application of various classifications and labels.[17] It then becomes essential to disciplinary techniques and control that individuals accept and internalize the characterizations those labels and classifications represent.

Once people are gathered into designated populations, either by institutional walls – or the intermediate step of restriction to particular areas by social pressures – or with labels, and normalizing discipline is applied, the basic operant principle, as mentioned earlier, is an ancient one. That principle is that if people are made to behave in certain ways for long enough, and under the right conditions, those ways of behaving will become habitual to them. The deeper result is that in becoming habitual, the inculcated ways of behaving reshape and redefine individuals, altering their self-perceptions, and, in effect, modifying *who they are*. But if Foucault shows us anything, it is that inculcating ways of behaving in people, and getting them to adopt new conceptions of who they are and how they should act, is anything but straightforward.

The trouble is that normalization is vulnerable to unpredictability in two different ways. Both have to do with the application of behaviour-modifying discipline, but one has to do with power relations while the other has to do with ethical effort. The first way unpredictability is introduced begins with the fact that discipline is always applied to serve a particular institution's objectives. However, the development of objectives, and the planning of how to achieve them, both occur in an environment of power relations, just as does the implementation of those plans. This means that power relations condition or modify development and planning, just as they condition or modify implementation, so institutional structuring and discipline actually achieve something rather different than the avowed objectives. That is, planners have an objective, and they set out to formulate ways to achieve it. But in the process, the objective may be subtly or not so subtly changed by the power relations influencing its articulation and the planning for its achievement. The objective actually served by the resulting plans, then, may differ significantly from its initial description, a description that most likely will be retained and not questioned. For instance, as Foucault explores in *Discipline and Punish*, the avowed objective of penal reforms was to humanize the treatment of inmates, but what was done in fact greatly increased penal institutions' control of inmates.

Another point that needs to be made about power relations is that discipline is always applied in the context of local power relations, which will differ from those of the broader context in which objectives are developed and plans to achieve them are worked out. This means that the actions done by those applying discipline – the issuing of orders, the drawing up of schedules, observation, examination, assessment, counselling, and so on – invariably will have unexpected consequences from the perspective of planners. This is because other past and present actions occurring in particular contexts condition even the most punctilious application of discipline. For instance, the same discipline technique applied in two institutions having somewhat different histories will yield different results. The work ethos and actual situation of one ward or hospital will differ enough from another's that a new rule imposed on both will have different results in each. There will be unavoidable differences, for instance, in how carefully the rule is administered, how rigorously it is adhered to, whether it is welcomed or resented, and how it impacts on other rules and prohibitions. Think again of the different responses to patients being required to pay for tests by physicians working in a hospital in an affluent community, and those working in an economically depressed neighbourhood.

The second way unpredictability is introduced into normalization is by how individuals respond to discipline. Their responses are conditioned or even determined not only by how others around them act, but also by how they themselves feel they should act. How they feel they should act is a complex function of their histories, who they take themselves to be, how acting in a particular manner conforms with or goes against that self-image, who they aspire to be, and how particular actions enhance or detract from that goal. Of course, how they do act is conditioned by power relations, as noted, but the impetus to act in a particular way sometimes arises from within individuals rather than from external influences. As a consequence, discipline's results differ even more from those intended. However sophisticated the planning and implementation of discipline techniques may be, the actual results of their application will be vector products of the many influences active in the context of power relations in which they are applied, and of how the disciplined individuals respond. But there is still more, because the actual results of the application of discipline affect the disciplining institution in various ways. The interaction between a disciplining institution, those who do the disciplining, and those who are disciplined is dynamic and reciprocal.

Most of the foregoing can be briefly put in the following way. The discipline that an institution applies at any given time is conditioned and shaped, and its results largely determined, by several factors. These are:

- The power relations in which objectives are developed
- The power relations in which attainment of those objectives is planned
- The power relations in which the plans are implemented
- The power relations in which individuals are disciplined
- Disciplined individuals' ethical efforts or attempts at self-determination

These general points can be translated into more specific terms having to do expressly with health care as follows. Health care's character and results are determined by:

- The power relations in which federal and provincial objectives and policies (e.g., universal access) are developed
- The power relations in which health care management is designed
- The power relations in which health care management is enacted
- The power relations in which health care is delivered and received
- How individuals actually deliver or respond to treatment

What introduction of power relations and ethics provides, over more familiar thinking and terminology, is a way of catching up much that presently is dismissed or ignored as human quirks and foibles that are beyond the reach of productive analysis. A grasp of the roles of power relations and ethical effort enables productive analysis of what otherwise looks too nebulous and unstructured to consider usefully. What we might otherwise take as people acting on whims or for unfathomable reasons looks more tractable when we think systematically in terms of their actions being constrained by the actions of others and by their own attempts at self-determination. This is not to say that Foucauldian power relations and ethics will enable us to purge health care of unpredictability. But it is to say that they will enable better understanding of that unpredictability, and so make possible more effective responses to things going wrong.

TAKING STOCK

A great deal needs to be said about health care in the chapters that follow. The foregoing is intended to provide a theoretical grounding for what we say about health care. However, there is a fine line between grounding what we say about health care on Foucault's genealogy and ethics, and turning discussion of health care and its present crisis into an academic exercise. We do not want to do the latter. The point of our necessarily sketchy outline of Foucault's genealogical and ethical ideas is to support our claim that health care's ills are some of them intrinsic to the system. Foucault's views enable us to say how health care's problems go beyond planning mistakes, policy errors, and management difficulties. We want to show how health care's problems are in part generated *by health care itself*, regardless of how ably planned and run, and we need Foucault's ideas to break through the current obsession with construing all problems as conventional management problems. Some problems are not conventional management problems; they do not admit of resolution by application of newer or better techniques. Some problems are inherent in enterprises and need to be allowed for because they cannot be fixed.

Reviews of health care's problems abound. Often it seems that there is little else in media coverage and political, professional, and scholarly discussion of health care. But reviewing health care's problems proves a very different and much more productive exercise when the review is conducted in light of how some of those problems are inherent to the enterprise, as opposed to being merely unforeseen glitches. The worrying reports, surveys, statistics, and anecdotes that only depress and concern us prove to be useful and enlightening when they are considered with an eye to what can be fixed and what can only be understood and allowed for. In essence, looking at health care's problems from a Foucauldian perspective, alive to the role of power relations and efforts at self-determination, enables recognition of management limitations and of how some of what goes wrong does so for reasons that are not amenable to application of corporate-model management techniques. If nothing else, this can prevent fruitless and expensive efforts to fix what cannot be fixed. Understanding health care in terms of genealogy and Foucauldian ethics provides the means to, first, comprehend how things go wrong, and second, appreciate what can be usefully changed and what can only be worked with or around.

Fortunately, what Foucault offers can be put in simpler language for our purposes, so long as we keep in mind that a great deal underlies our glosses. The basic move here is to distinguish among three different sorts of behavioural determinants. First, there are what we will call *institutional influences*. These primarily are the procedural rules that institutions impose on their agents and clients. However, along with specific directives, we also include under the "institutional influences" rubric the foundational principles and constitutive canons that define particular institutions. Second, there are what we will call *contextual influences*. These are what Foucault focuses on in his genealogical analysis of power relations. It should be kept in mind that he sees institutional influences as basically products or constructs of contextual influences. Contextual influences are determinants of behaviour in the sense that they are how the actions of others constrain given individuals' actions. Unlike explicit institutional influences, contextual influences largely are implicit or tacit. They are unspoken because they are not directives; they are purely relational influences on behaviour. Contextual influences are power relations; they are actions constraining actions. Third, there are what we will call internal or *subjective influences*. These are behavioural determinants that have sources internal to individuals, in that they are all the influences on individuals' behaviour that arise from personal history and efforts to be a certain sort of person. Subjective influences are what Foucauldian ethics are all about. We include internal or subjective influences that are not as reflective as are deliberate attempts at self-determination, though we do not want to lump all manner of psychological determinants of behaviour under the "subjective influences." For instance, in our stethoscope example, the young doctor who wears her stethoscope on rounds does so in largely unconscious emulation of her mentor, whereas in treating patients in certain ways she emulates her mentor in a knowing and deliberate way.

Given the foregoing rubrics, we can say that what we think is new in our application of Foucault's ideas to health care is that subjective influences have to be factored into any analysis of contextual influences. It is not enough to offer genealogical analyses of power relations in health care – or penality or any other institutional system. Ethical analyses must complement genealogical analyses. An analysis

of health care requires recognition of how subjective influences condition contextual influences. That is, trying to understand how health
care's agents' and clients' actions influence others' actions requires
understanding how each agent's or client's actions are shaped by
their ethical efforts, in Foucault's proprietary sense of "ethical." In
short, how individuals' self-determinative impulses and intentions
mould and direct their actions is as important as how those actions
are constrained by others' actions. Only in this way can we really
understand how complex human interactions proceed in institutional
settings or, in our terms, environments of institutional influences. The
modification of proactive and reactive actions by self-determinative
influences is integral to how individuals act, and so to how their
actions constrain others' actions.

Distinguishing among institutional, contextual, and subjective
influences lets us make our general point succinctly: *effective management techniques must acknowledge that contextual and subjective influences
generate problems that are intrinsic to any institutional enterprise.* Present
management techniques automatically cast institutional problems as
technical problems; that is, management techniques construe and
address problems as issues that can be resolved with better assessment and planning, better resources, better procedures, better administration, and so on. As we hope to show, in the case of health care,
this approach is not good enough.

CHAPTER THREE

Health Care and Chaos

Assessing how health care works and fails to work is an *analytic* exercise; it is a matter of looking at a whole and seeing how its parts work or fail to work. But designing or – more important for us – reforming a health care system, is not an analytic exercise; it is a *synthesizing* exercise and so vastly harder to achieve successfully. The problem is that in synthesizing we have to begin with various elements or components and put them together in a way that will ensure that each works as it is supposed to work when it is integrated into a dynamic whole. Clearly, an attempted synthesis cannot succeed if a component that is supposed to perform in one way actually performs differently when it interacts with other components. And obviously, the more components there are, the greater are the chances that their interaction will yield unexpected results. In some cases, that possibility all but precludes that we will be able to predict with any conviction how a given component will function in conjunction with others. Health care has a very large number of human and non-human components or variables. In addition, its human components are changeable. Each is individually prone to "internal" change, and how each functions as a component of health care also changes, as outlined in the previous chapter, depending on how others affect and work with him or her. It is this unpredictability that ensures that not even the most inspired planning and meticulous management can be assured of achieving intended objectives. Health care's complexity arises both from the number of its components and from the changeable character of some of those components. This means that its unpredictability is not only a function of things going wrong, it is in part a function of its very nature.

In this chapter we have to look at health care's complexity from two different perspectives. The first has to do with the nature of complex systems; the second has to do with the behaviour of some of health care's components, namely, the people who serve it and whom it serves. We begin by discussing the abstract issue of system complexity and unpredictability or "chaos." We then return to Foucault to discuss health care's agents' and clients' ethical efforts. The point is to better understand health care's complexity, and how that complexity is greatly enlarged by the behaviour of health care's human components. The objective is to appreciate the magnitude of health care's unpredictability, because such appreciation is a necessary condition of effective, productive reform.

ANALYSIS AND SYNTHESIS

The issue of the difficulty with synthesis is clearly evident in science, especially in the biological sciences. Speaking of efforts at "interlocking ... the biological disciplines," Edward O. Wilson remarks that it is "vastly more difficult" to synthesize than to analyze. He points out that "[t]he greatest obstacle to consilience [unification] by synthesis ... is the exponential increase in complexity encountered during the upward progress through levels of organization."[1] In the case of the biological sciences, analyzing an organism down to its molecular components is difficult but relatively straightforward; starting with molecular components and trying to determine the organism they might compose is immensely more difficult. Even if we move up the scale from microcomponents to macro ones, things are not significantly better.[2] Wilson gives an example of a small tract of land isolated by flooding. The isolation of the tract removed a single predator from it, and that resulted in huge and unpredictable changes to its ecology.[3] Trying to predict those changes, on the basis of information or hypotheses about the removal of a single predator, would have met with limited success. We might have predicted the effects on the local fauna, for instance, of an increase in the population of the predator's prey, but likely not the effects to local flora. The problem of successfully working our way up from molecular components to organisms, or from ecological elements to ecosystems, is enormous. Wilson thinks that "[t]he greatest challenge today, not just in cell biology and ecology but in all of science, is the accurate and complete description of complex systems." He adds that while "[s]cientists have broken down many kinds of systems," the challenge they face now "is to reassemble them, at least in mathematical models that capture the key properties of the entire ensembles."[4]

However, while immensely difficult, "complete description of complex systems" in science is possible, even if only in principle. But in health care, the fact that some of health care's components are malleable, impressionable individuals means that complete description is not possible in practice or in principle. This is why health care's "assembly" in mathematical or statistical models is so risky a practice and so limited in its scope of possible success. Initiating a health care system, or reforming one, is an exercise in synthesis, not analysis, and however difficult synthesis is in science, successful synthesis is effectively precluded in health care because of its malleable human components. Therefore, anticipating the consequences of introducing changes is not just an immensely complex task, it is one that cannot be successfully done – certainly not with our present knowledge and techniques. Unfortunately, those who are concerned to reform health care proceed as if unaware of the difference between analysis and synthesis. They seem quite confident that analysis of the existing institution is enough to provide a sound basis for making improvements. But analysis is not enough; changes made on the basis of analysis will have limited success, at best, and could have disastrously counterproductive results. To say how and why, we have to expand on the foregoing. We begin with some remarks about natural systems.

VARIABLES AND PREDICTABILITY

Chaos theory is the "branch of mathematics used to deal with chaotic systems."[5] Chaos theorists deal with "dynamical systems" that are both quantifiable and deterministic in the sense of being bound by physical laws. The simplest dynamical systems are mechanical ones, and they are deterministic in a readily grasped way: a mechanical device has a set number of possible states and predictable and retrodictable transitions from one state to another. More complex dynamical systems are chemical reactions and planetary motion. In these, the possible states and transitions of the system increase exponentially. A still more complex dynamical system is the weather. As a system's complexity and variables increase, so does the presence of "chaos" or unpredictability. However, a chaotic system is not truly erratic; that is, it does not defy physical laws. A chaotic system is one that is complex enough that even very small changes in its many variables result in unpredictable consequences from our point of view. Characterization of a system as chaotic is an epistemological move. That is, to characterize a dynamical system as chaotic is not to say that it is unpredictable "in the order of being" or in itself as a series of physical events. It is to say that the system is unpredictable "in the order of knowledge," or in terms of our comprehension of it, due to the number of its variables and to the limits on our ability to identify and track those variables. The weather is a case in point. To predict weather accurately, we would need to know the air pressure, humidity, and temperature of every significant volume – say, every square mile – of Earth's atmosphere. We would also have to constantly update that knowledge. In other words, we would have to map atmospheric states and changes exhaustively and continuously, which we clearly cannot do. The weather is a chaotic dynamical system because its variables and state transitions, despite being bound by physical laws, outstrip our ability to map them with the requisite accuracy.

The relevance of chaotic dynamical systems here is that some systems are intrinsically chaotic, in the epistemological sense or our comprehension of them, because of the number of their variables and possible state transitions. Chaotic systems are so complex that we cannot fully determine and describe their present states, therefore we cannot accurately predict their future states nor retrodict their past states. The import of this in the present context is two fold: first, our predictions and expectations regarding some systems can only be of a quite general sort and so are useful only at the macro level. Second, and most important, when our predictions go awry, and our expectations are not met, the reasons may be intrinsic to the system as opposed to being extraneous. In short, when something goes wrong in a complex system, we cannot always look to external causes. Sometimes we must accept that things go wrong because of a system's structure and development, and not because something outside the system interfered with its workings.

The parallel we are drawing between chaotic systems and health care is designed to show that when things go wrong in health care, it is not always because of mistakes, ignorance, and so on. Sometimes things work out as they do because of health care's inherent nature, in the sense that its components behave in ways that are unpredictable, not because of error or ignorance, but because of how the system bears on each of them. Therefore, what goes wrong cannot always be fixed with techniques that presuppose that problems are due to interference with the system, as opposed to being due to something about the system itself. Health care, viewed as a system, has more than enough "variables" to be chaotic in the technical sense, and aside from sheer numbers, health care has various sorts of variables or components. There are its procedures, drugs, equipment, economics, demographics, sites, and so on. Each of these may vary in different ways. For instance, with respect to drugs and procedures, a promising pill's effectiveness quite unexpectedly may be diminished if it happens to be taken with grapefruit juice instead of water; a bypass surgery procedure surprisingly may permanently impede memory function by reducing blood flow to the brain.[6] But what most makes health care intrinsically unpredictable are its *people*. Health care's most important variables or components are its managers, its practitioners, and its patients – or, from a Foucauldian perspective, their actions.[7] It is the complex behaviour of its human components that raises health care's unpredictability to a level that seems increasingly beyond our capacity to manage.

Health care's most worrying unpredictability is due to the interactions of its human components and to their individual efforts. To refer to this higher order of "chaos" or complexity, we borrow – and modify – a term from what is called "action morphicity" theory as developed by Harry Collins and Martin Kusch.[8] The term we borrow is "polymorphic" (literally, "many-shaped"), which Collins and Kusch use to describe how humans behave when "they draw on their understanding of their society."[9] The term is used to contrast with mechanical behaviour. Basically the difference is that between acting in a reflective way and acting in a robot-like manner. Our adoption of the term is intended to convey two things. The first is that humans are defined by polymorphic action, not just in that they act in ways that "draw on their understanding of their society," but that their actions are determined by the influence of others on them – in other words, by power relations. Second, a system having human beings as components is polymorphic in that its states and transitions, as a system, are in part determined by the complex interactions of individuals acting polymorphically. We feel this term captures what is special about health care viewed as a system, which is that however chaotic it may be in virtue of the number and behaviour of its non-human variables, it is far more chaotic or unpredictable in virtue of the behaviour of its human variables. Health care is polymorphic in both of these two ways, and hence is doubly chaotic and unpredictable in nature.

The best we can do by way of tracking a polymorphic system's variables and transition states is the same as what we do with chaotic systems like the weather. That is, we can develop statistical bases for predictions even though we know they will prove even more uncertain than those we produce about systems like the weather. Yet despite this, management of health care, and more recently medical practice itself, are increasingly and, it seems, uncritically dependent on statistical predictions. Our point is not, of course, that statistical models and the predictions they ground are of no use. They clearly are of use. The trouble is that while of use at the macro level, which is where statistics belong, application of statistical models and predictions at the micro level is fraught with danger. In the delivery of health care, no physician can treat a patient on the basis of averages. As for health care management, our example about the counterproductive schedule illustrates the sort of problem that can occur with uncritical reliance on statistics.

The main problem we see is that, as we have been stressing, health care's agents and clients are malleable. They are susceptible to change because of how they are classified, the duties they are assigned, the expectations they must meet, how other health care agents and clients behave, and how they individually are treated. Therefore, health care does not involve just so many agents and clients; each one of them is constantly changed to some degree by how health care is managed, practised, and received. Agents' and clients' behaviour, then, will vary significantly in different contexts and at different times. So however carefully planned and managed it may be, health care generates unpredictability. It does so by continually reshaping those who manage it, those who provide it, and those who use it. To make things worse, not only does health care change its agents and clients, each of them is, to some extent, trying to change him- or herself, thus introducing even more unpredictability.

Health care being a polymorphic system means that statistical models of health care, or of some of its aspects, are problematic in their applicability. As in the case of models of other complex systems, such as of the weather, statistical models in health care, and the projections they support, are only representations. If the models

served only an analytic purpose, that is, if statistics were used to
show how things developed during past periods for which we have
reliable data, or to show how things currently stand in the whole or
some aspect of health care, things would be much simpler. But statistical models are widely used for synthesizing purposes in health
care management and policy development. That is, they are used to
base projections of future situations on the basis of past and current
situations, and so to ground and justify decisions. For instance, statistical models are used to justify cost cutting by, say, curtailing surgical procedures that present data indicate are being increasingly
supplanted by pharmacological treatment. However, such data in
fact may represent current fashion more than the superior effectiveness of medication over surgery in some application. The trouble is
that models always require interpretation, and some require more
than others. Models are problematic even in the sciences. Speaking
of models in science, Wilson comments on the basic problem in connection with biologists who develop algorithms to advance their
syntheses of various phenomena. When an algorithm yields positive
results, the question that arises is how biologists

know that nature's algorithms are the same as their own, or even close.
Many procedures may be false and yet produce an approximately correct
answer ... To see this point clearly, think of a blossom in a painting rendered
photographic in detail ... From a distance we might ... confuse the image
with the real thing. But the algorithms that created it are radically different.
Its microscopic elements are flakes of paint instead of chromosomes and cells
... How do theoreticians know that their ... simulations are not just the
paintings of flowers?[10]

Models are, after all, just that: models. They claim to represent
realities that may be very different from the models even when there
seems to be conformity between model and reality. The fact is that
the conformity may be only apparent; it may be superficial, merely
a matter of appearances. This is not to say that statistical models are
not useful; they clearly are and we often construct them correctly. But
consider that the facts never support only one model. We know
from science that several incommensurable theories may fit the facts.
This is even truer of models. Numerous models may fit the facts. Our
choices among models, like our choices among theories, are not made
purely on the basis of the models' or theories' adequacy to the data

or facts. Elegance plays a major role in choosing among theories, as it does in choosing among models. History and tradition also play their roles. Recently we have learned that gender plays a highly consequential role.[11] In any case, our point here is that the more complex the phenomenon modelled, the more problematic the model. However, there is a less obvious point that also needs to be made, one with special relevance to health care management and reform.

As noted, models are models. However, this is sometimes lost sight of in enterprises involving complex management techniques. That is, models are sometimes mistaken for the realities they model. This does not happen in a simple way; it is not just a matter of confusing one thing for another. It happens when use of and reliance on a model in effect collapse the distance between the model and the reality. Somewhat different, but of great significance to health care, is that, as we consider below, there is a great danger that a model may be misconstrued as a management plan. One way this can happen is when a model, originally intended to explore or investigate certain suspected tendencies or trends, is increasingly misused to justify planning decisions. Here, rather than a model being confused with what it models, a model that portrays a past, or at best a present, reality is confused with directions for establishing a new or future reality.

Health care is extremely complex, yet health care planners, reformers, and managers rely heavily on models. The role of statistical and other models in health care planning, management, and reform has grown markedly in the last two or three decades. Somewhat paradoxically, that growth has not been slowed by how health care's unpredictability regularly demonstrates itself to be even greater than that of the most chaotic physical systems.

Health care's unpredictability, and so the problematic nature of its statistical and predictive models, is due primarily to the fact that its agents and clients are not stable elements in the system. They are unpredictably changed by the system itself, and so behave unpredictably. They thus render the system chaotic in a way that is not a result of the system's own structure or sheer number of variables. Examples of how health care's human variables change are, to name just three, managers dealing with persistent resource shortages who become unresponsive to special needs, practitioners faced with overly heavy caseloads who start to cut corners, and patients enduring long waiting periods who begin to exaggerate their symptoms. But what these examples bring out is that not only do health care's agents and clients behave irregularly, from a system planner's perspective, their unpredictable behaviour in turn affects the system. Unresponsive managers, corner-cutting practitioners, and symptom-exaggerating patients in various ways impede health care management and treatment, and invariably raise costs. These examples, though, are of reactive or responsive behaviour. That is, they are examples of behaviour prompted by what we are calling institutional influences. But agents' and clients' actions are not only affected by how the health care system bears on them. Their actions are also constrained by the behaviour of those they work for, those they work with, those they treat, and those who treat them – in other words, by what we are calling contextual influences or what Foucault calls power relations. But however complicated things may be, with respect to institutional and contextual influences, they are further complicated by subjective influences. That is, agents and clients are not only affected by various directives and the actions of those around them, they are also engaged in a continuing process of self-definition or self-determination. That is, each individual is, to a greater or lesser extent, trying to be a certain person. Each one's behaviour, then, is shaped not only by others' actions, but by subjective values, fears, inclinations, and, in particular, their efforts to be the person they feel they are and want to be. This is the topic we pursue in the next section.

In the previous chapter we indicated how the unpredictable results of health care's influences on its agents and clients are multiplied by the haphazard consequences of human interactions, that is, by contextual influences or power relations. In this chapter we have tried to show how health care is an intrinsically unpredictable system. To that end we have drawn a parallel between health care and chaotic dynamical systems. The parallel is adequate to demonstrating how health care's agents and clients behave unpredictably as the human components of health care viewed as a system. This would suffice to show that, at least in degree, health care is a very special, if not unique, chaotic system. But the parallel drawn falls short of showing how the unpredictability of health care's agents' and clients' behaviour goes beyond the interactive influences we have inventoried. We also need to clarify how agents' and clients' own self-defining efforts greatly augment the unpredictability that is due to their interaction. Part of the importance of doing so is that while health care's agents and clients can be seen as interacting components or variables of a chaotic system, they make health care unpredictable in a way that has no parallel in the physical world. As human beings, health care's agents and clients behave in ways that are prompted by purely internal factors quite unlike anything found in the physical environment.

"ETHICS"

It may seem odd to consider what Foucault conceives to be ethics in connection with chaotic systems and unpredictability. However, as indicated, Foucauldian ethics are about how individuals attempt to determine their own behaviour. The connection to health care's unpredictability is that, as components of the health care system, the unpredictability resulting from individuals' Foucauldian ethical behaviour is of major significance. If individuals are inevitably engaged in self-defining projects that affect how they behave, their roles as components of the health care system clearly will be affected. Foucauldian ethics help us to understand how health care's agents' and clients' efforts at self-determination affect their behaviour. The point of gaining this understanding is less to achieve better predictions than it is to appreciate the inescapability of disruptive pressures on the workings of health care. What is most important, in the present context, is not so much what individuals actually do; rather, it is that they are prone to do things for reasons that others usually are neither privy to nor can easily anticipate. That is what matters here, that human beings act in unexpected ways, not only because of the power relations they find themselves in, but for their own reasons.

Health care's agents and clients, then, behave as they do only partly because of institutional influences or how health care requires them to behave, and only partly because of contextual influences or interaction with others. They also behave as they do partly because of subjective influences or internal prompting. The unpredictability of health care's agents' and clients' behaviour, therefore, arises from a dynamic fusion of imposed duties and expectations, the impact of their peers' actions, and their own fears and aspirations. Each of these factors contributes to the end result in a complicated way. Against the backdrop of health care's institutional influences, contextual influences condition compliance with imposed duties and expectations in ways that may result in unanticipated behaviour and consequences. Subjective influences then further condition and skew both compliance with institutional influences and contextual influences. The outcome is unpredictable behaviour. We also need to remember that the unpredictable behaviour adds significantly to the contextual influences on others.

Some simple instances of these complex interactions are the following. Compliance with a directive on informing patients about treatment side effects, for instance, may be conditioned by how things are done in a particular ward. The effect is that perhaps patients are given too much detail in one ward, too little detail in another. In the one case, patients may be confused; in the other, patients may be inadvertently misinformed. The particular reasons why too little or too much information is given are very varied. For instance, gender is often an issue here. Some male, and even a few female, physicians may unwittingly or even consciously take it for granted that female patients are unlikely to understand certain points about treatment or side effects that male patients are likelier to appreciate. Age is also often an issue. Male and female physicians, nurses, and other providers regularly assume that elderly patients will not understand much of what they might be told about treatment and side effects. In any case, the results actually achieved by the directive will be different than those intended. Again, compliance with a conservative directive on sedative dosages, say, may conflict with physicians' own experience, resulting in their regularly prescribing and justifying higher doses, and effectively circumventing the directive. In such cases, not only is the directive circumvented, if the practice comes to be consistent and fairly widespread, administration directives will be paid less and less attention, thus establishing counterproductive contextual influences. Another sort of case is where a change in duties and expectations, such as the imposition of a new schedule, prompts resentment and counterproductive, excessively rigid compliance, as in our earlier example. In addition, all of these problematic responses also add to contextual influences in that they establish local precedents for responding to unwelcome administrative changes.

As discussed above, in power relations every person is both a subjective and a subjected identity. To be a subject is to be a subjugated individual; it is to be "subject to someone else by control and dependence." To be a subject also is to have one's identity defined "by a conscience or self–knowledge."[12] Note that Foucault says "conscience," not "consciousness" or "self-awareness." This is because he is not referring only to self-awareness; he is referring to value-conditioned self-awareness. His understanding of what it is to be a subject of experience is thoroughly normative. To be a subject is not just to be aware of the world and of oneself; it is to be aware of the world and of oneself in value-laden and value-determined ways. We are defined, not by sheer awareness, but by a subjectivity that is in part constituted by likes and dislikes, fears and desires, yearnings and dreads. We cannot achieve neutral perception of ourselves or the world around us. Our self-awareness is always conditioned by who we think we are, who we are afraid we are, who we want to be, and especially by whom others treat us as being. In his genealogical works, primarily *Discipline and Punish* and the first volume of *The History of Sexuality*, Foucault is concerned with how power relations mould subjects. His focus is on how an individual, as a subject of experience, is shaped by being governed, by being disciplined. "What does a discipline do? It shapes individuals – neither with nor without their consent."[13] Genealogically conceived, the subject of experience, the subjective identity, is a *product* of power relations. In other words, in genealogy, the subjugated individual is primary; the subjective individual is secondary because it is a product of how the subjected individual is regulated and disciplined. But in his ethics, Foucault reverses the relational priority, focusing on the subjective identity, on the subjective individual engaged in self-creation and only secondarily subjugated by externally imposed moral codes, regulations, disciplines, and practices.

Traditional ethics are about our relationships with others and our obligations to them – or to the state or to God. As indicated earlier, contrary to this familiar sense of "ethics," Foucault's ethics are not about others but about "the self's relationship to itself."[14] They are about how we "transform" and "modify" ourselves "to attain a certain state of perfection."[15] The Foucauldian ethical subject is not one primarily concerned with obligations to family, friends, or society, but one who tries to make him- or herself into a person who instantiates certain values. The basic idea is the Nietzschean one of self-creation. This is the idea that each of us should remake ourselves so that we, and our lives are, literally, works of art, that is, the products of deliberate choice and purposeful self-determination. This is another place gender becomes important, because it is only since feminist work began to make an impact on the general public that many women began to realize that they need not accept many roles traditionally assigned to them and thus became Foucauldian ethical subjects. This development is highly significant to health care, because of the very high percentage of health care providers who are women.

Probably only a few engage in self-creation in a deliberate and holistic way, but we are all Foucauldian ethical subjects to the extent that our past experience, aspirations, and disappointments make us try to do some things and not others, and to do what we do in certain ways or in a certain "style." This means that our reactions to control and regulation are complicated by how doing or not doing a huge range of things affects our perception of ourselves, our self-image, and whether what is required of us harmonizes with or hampers our self-determinative efforts.

To flesh out the foregoing, a bit more must be said about Foucauldian ethics; in particular, it is necessary to sketch how his ethics consist of four elements:

- "Ethical substance," or what Ian Hacking calls the "the sheer stuff you worry about if you are a moral agent"[16]
- "The mode of subjection," or how "the individual establishes his relation to the rule" – in essence, the recognition of moral principles and responsibility
- "Ethical work," or what "one performs on oneself" to comply with moral codes and "to transform oneself" into the ethical subject one aspires to be
- The "telos," or the idealized ethical subject one strives to become[17]

Of these, what concern us are the "mode of subjection," or how individuals relate themselves to regulations, and the "telos," or the persons individuals are trying to become. These two elements bear directly on health care management because they often are at odds with one another, leading to the need to make various sorts of on-the-job compromises, as when complying with some regulation runs counter to acting as one is inclined or aspires to act. This is especially true where regulations counter individuals' partialities, and do so in emotionally charged situations. For instance, hospital regulations may specify ways of dealing with do-not-resuscitate orders that some physicians find in conflict with their own experience with terminal cases or their moral compunctions. They then may deal with do-not-resuscitate orders in ways that effectively subvert policy and also influence others in unproductive ways. Again, operating-room nurses may have moral compunctions about assisting with partial-birth abortions and do so in ways that raise their own and possibly others' stress levels.

These examples indicate the importance of understanding that what we are calling subjective influences, or Foucauldian ethics, do not encompass only grand efforts to remake oneself. Something as simple as quitting smoking is an instance of acting in a way determined by subjective influences, and it can have important consequences. For instance, a physician might choose to not attend a staff meeting because of concern that others will be smoking and that early in his or her attempt to quit smoking, he or she will lack the resolve to not smoke when others do. The physician's absence could have important repercussions on others' behaviour. Due to being absent, the physician may fail to have important input to a weighty discussion; again, others may interpret that absence as a sign of disaffection or estrangement. As in the case of genealogy, in Foucauldian ethics the main focus must be on what Hacking calls "tiny local events" that jointly determine much larger developments.[18] Whatever the intended results, and whether or not they are achieved, people's actions always have additional results to the extent that those actions bear on others in that nearly everything people do contributes to contextual influences or power relations affecting others – and themselves.

In summary, Foucauldian ethical efforts or subjective influences determine a significant part of what health care's agents and clients do. That is, a good deal of what individuals do is done in ways that meet their internal expectations about what is proper action, under the circumstances, for the persons they take themselves to be or are trying to become. The young female doctor in our stethoscope example is internally motivated to emulate a physician she admires and who greatly influenced her. She does not see wearing her stethoscope on rounds as flaunting a badge of office, nor as marking herself off from nurses and other providers. If she thinks of it at all, she sees wearing the stethoscope as being like her mentor, perhaps as being a tiny bit more ready to check a patient, and she would consider it foolish for someone to think that she is symbolically asserting her position. The doctor's wearing her stethoscope, however, conflicts with others' expectations and perceptions, and so influences how they behave. In that way, the doctor's subjective influences, her Foucauldian ethical effort, contributes to the contextual influences or power relations influencing others' actions.

To close this chapter, we need to re-emphasize the crucial link between unpredictability or chaos, on the one hand, and subjective influences or ethical effort, on the other. This link is that subjective influences introduce a kind of unpredictability that augments systemic unpredictability in two different ways. First, subjective influences simply add to systemic unpredictability. That is, whatever unpredictability is generated by health care's many components is increased by the unpredictability generated by its agents and clients trying to go their own way. Second, the unpredictability generated by health care's components affects its agents and clients in ways that exacerbate subjective influences, thus increasing unpredictability. That is, when policies or management's directives result in unpredictable consequences, because of contextual influences or power relations, individuals are prompted to deal with those consequences in ways that more than likely introduce conflicts with their subjective influences. For example, the perception of a directive's ineffectiveness – as when the schedule in our earlier example proves counterproductive – forces individuals to deal with tensions and contradictions between institutional influences and contextual influences. How they do so invariably introduces more unpredictability, if only because different individuals will respond in different ways. Health care's systemic unpredictability, then, is not only augmented by subjective influences, it is compounded by what people do in striving for self-determination. The following is a case in point that nicely illustrates how subjective influences or Foucauldian ethical effort can affect an individual's own medical treatment and, eventually, both others' treatment and physicians' practices.

Statins are cholesterol-lowering drugs that are being increasingly used to treat and attempt to prevent cardiovascular disease. Basically, statins inhibit the liver's production of cholesterol. The liver needs cholesterol, so with production inhibited, it develops extra receptors that collect cholesterol from the bloodstream. In this way, statins reduce the level of cholesterol in the body and the buildup of cholesterol in the blood vessels. Statins were discovered in 1976, and their widespread use is relatively recent, so experience with long-term side effects is somewhat limited. This poses a potential problem, as some are so impressed with the results of statin therapy that they want the drug sold over the counter as a public health measure. These same supporters of statin therapy think people as young as in their thirties should take statins as preventive therapy.[19]

Statins now constitute a variable in health care, both insofar as they are used in treatment and in that some consider they should be used as preventive therapy. However, a question arises that seems obvious, even though it may be biochemically naive. The cholesterol the liver produces is of the HDL, or high-density, sort; the cholesterol the liver collects from the bloodstream when statins are used is of the LDL, or low-density, sort. This is partly why statins are so effective, because the cholesterol collected is the "bad" sort that accumulates in the blood vessels. But aside from statins' known side effects, such as muscle inflammation, what are the effects of the liver using significantly more LDLs than HDLS over a long period of time, if the liver is, so to speak, "designed" to use HDLS? The question could have important repercussions if a provincial government policy were adopted to prescribe statins, as a preventive measure, to people who show elevated cholesterol levels but no symptoms of cardiovascular disease. If having fifty-year-olds taking statins significantly reduces the number of sixty-year-olds needing treatment for cardiovascular disease, significant savings could be realized, and such a policy would look attractive to health care planners and managers. This is the point at which subjective influences enter the picture.[20]

A typical example is that of a fifty-two-year-old woman with elevated cholesterol, but no other cardiovascular problems, whose physician recommended statin therapy. She declined to take the drug, instead choosing to lower her cholesterol level through diet and exercise. "For me, it was almost a pride thing," she remarked, adding that she led a healthy lifestyle, was in good health, and had asked both herself and her physician, "Why should I have to take this pill?"[21] The answer could be that by doing so she would lower her cholesterol level significantly more than through diet and exercise, and at the same time be able to relax the demanding regimen she had imposed on herself. But what is important here is that the woman did see refusing statin therapy as "a pride thing." This is a clear instance of subjective influences determining someone's behaviour. Perhaps more important for our purposes it is an instance of someone who would be expected to avail herself of statins' efficacy refusing to do so. If a large number of people respond to proposed statin therapy in this way, the implemented preventive policy would not yield the expected savings regardless of the drug's effectiveness. Moreover, of those choosing not to take statins, likely only a few would successfully lower their cholesterol levels through exercise and diet. The other side of the coin is that those taking statins might be lulled into complacency and increase their intake of fats as well as reduce their exercise, thereby neutralizing the drug's benefits. In that case, the preventive therapy policy would have little or no effect, at best, and at worst prove counterproductive.

The determining of behaviour by subjective influences, then, adds significantly to health care's unpredictability as a system by increasing agents' and clients' unanticipated responses. It also compounds health care's unpredictability because behaviour determined by subjective influences aggravates contextual influences.

This and previous chapters are intended to provide a theoretical backdrop for the more empirical and politically nuanced discussion of health care that follows in part 2 of this book. As some of the foregoing material is difficult, repetition has been necessary, the complex has been simplified, and much that demands lengthy discussion has been glossed over. But as noted earlier, we did not want exposition of our theoretical base to turn into an academic exercise; the point is to ground our analysis of health care's special problems. To proceed, we offer in the next and last chapter in this part a summary restatement of the main points covered thus far to make clearer how they apply to the discussion of health care that follows in part 2.

CHAPTER FOUR

Chaos, Power, and Ethics

In the preceding chapters we have considered how health care's human components – its agents and clients – may not behave as expected or directed to behave because of contextual influences and/or subjective influences or, in Foucauldian terminology, because of power relations and/or ethical effort. What they actually do and how they do it is only partly determined by what they are told to do or are supposed to do. Their behaviour also is partly determined by how others' actions influence their own actions, and by how they feel they need to act to comply with their own internal imperatives. The result is that as components of a complex system, people raise system unpredictability to a level well above that of even the most complex physical system. And while this is true of any complex system in which human beings interact, we maintain that it is especially true of health care. The basic reason is that the stakes – people's well-being – are very high, and the attendant responsibilities and stresses are equally high.

However, it must not be assumed that the unpredictable behaviour that concerns us is unusual or bizarre behaviour. The sort of unpredictability that most concerns us is not aberrant behaviour due to perversity or pathology. What concerns us has less to do with unforeseen departures from established routines than it does with how routines actually are carried out. The doing of something peculiar, or the not doing of something required, are relatively rare cases in health care, and there are established procedures to deal with odd, irresponsible, or insubordinate behaviour. Additionally, and most important, is that when these lapses do occur, they are evident to managers and peers, and the damage done usually can be set right or contained.

What is more dangerous to health care as a complex system is unpredictable behaviour that is not evident but is nonetheless disruptive. This consists of people responding to directives and expectations in counterproductive ways that compromise or undermine intended results and objectives. For instance, in our schedule example in chapter 2, compliance by the hospital's physicians with the new schedule actually defeats the schedule's purpose because the physicians not only spend less time with patients, they see fewer patients. As sketched in the example, resentment of the imposed schedule leads the physicians to stop working the longer hours they previously worked and did not report. But the consequences of their actions will not be evident for some time, and even when those consequences do become evident, they potentially will be attributed to other causes in retrospective analyses. The rise in teenage pregnancies, say, might be blamed, not on the hospital's physicians ceasing to counsel patients, but on increased use of drugs or greater promiscuity.

There are subtler and ultimately more damaging instances of how unpredictable behaviour damages a complex system. In fact, the more subtly agent and client behaviour fails to meet expectations, the more dangerous for the system. The obvious reason is that managers may remain unaware for some time that anything is amiss. The less obvious reason is that some kinds of unpredictable behaviour are cumulative in their feedback on the system. If enough compromises are made in dealing with an unpopular directive or implemented policy, the contextual influences generated preclude any possibility of the directive's or policy's aims being achieved. A further complication is that it may be some time before reliable statistics become available that show the directive's or policy's failure. In the meantime, a broad implemented policy or local directive intended to cut costs is at best only partially successful and is being rendered progressively less so. Cases of this sort seem particularly characteristic of health maintenance organizations in the United States. For instance, physicians are restricted from informing patients about the availability of tests and treatments that are both expensive and have a low level of statistical success. But physicians wanting to inform their patients about such treatments or tests, perhaps because their experience runs counter to the statistics, regularly circumvent the restrictions. For example, they can comply with the restrictions by not explicitly informing patients about a particular test or treatment but refer them to articles or Web sites dealing with their afflictions and discussing the tests or treatments. Such circumvention often is effectively augmented by the relatively new phenomenon of pharmaceutical companies advertising directly to consumers.[1]

The basic point here is that health care poses a possibly unique case with respect to the nature and extent of its complexity because it has both human and non-human variables, and its human components are subject to extraordinary pressures. Health care certainly meets the requirements to be a chaotic system in the sense that it is complex enough to generate unpredictability in an intrinsic way due to the number of its variables and the diversity of their interactions. The import of this, as we have stressed, is that health care's difficulties are not due only to extrinsic factors such as error, ignorance, chance events, and so on. Its variables are sufficiently numerous and diverse to ensure that, due to how even very small changes in those variables work their way through the system, we cannot accurately predict system-level consequences of initiatives or changes. The fact that only some of health care's variables are like the variables of chaotic physical systems, such as the weather, that are governed by physical laws means that systemic unpredictability has two dimensions: sheer complexity of physical interactions and consequences, and inherently unpredictable behaviour. Unlike variables that are directly caused to behave as they do, health care's agents and clients may and do behave in ways other than how they are told to behave or can reasonably be expected to behave. Moreover, even when they behave as they are told to behave, they may do so in ways that have different consequences than those intended.

Take just one example. The widely used drug ASA (aspirin) was brought into production for its analgesic effect. However, ASA subsequently turned out to have major implications for the treatment of coronary vascular disease, significantly altering the treatment of coronary vascular disease and having an unexpected positive effect on the cost of treating it. In this respect, unexpected results ensued from certain unforeseen physical interactions. But the unexpected side effects of ASA also had repercussions of a quite different sort than the beneficial ones of lowering costs and obviating some treatment of coronary vascular disease. While the health care system gained by the development of a cheap, effective new treatment, a new area of risk to patients' health was introduced precisely by the treatment's efficacy. As soon as news about ASA's vascular benefits was reported, individuals with high cholesterol levels or high blood pressure began to medicate themselves with ASA, rather than undergo the rigours of dieting or physical exercise. Others, without cholesterol or blood pressure problems, also medicated themselves as a preventive measure. In many cases self-medication led, on the one hand, to a rash of stomach ulcers and gastrointestinal bleeding, and, on the other, to the risk of more rapid onset of coronary illness because of delaying other necessary therapies. In addition, some individuals were made complacent, seeing an aspirin a day as a "magic bullet" and risking elevated cholesterol levels due to lack of care about their diet. The cumulative consequences of these factors likely negated or at least significantly reduced the cost benefits of ASA treatment. In this way, the unexpected consequences of physical-variable behaviour was augmented by the consequences of human-variable behaviour.

Individuals' efforts at self-determination modify how they act as agents and clients of the health care system. Aside from their doctors' recommendations and the advice of others, individuals may medicate themselves because of subjective influences such as self-perception of themselves as knowledgeable about contemporary medical developments. Individuals also modify their behaviour as agents and clients of health care because of what others around them are doing and have done, that is, because of contextual influences. The latter can run from quite unconscious to deliberate emulation or repudiation of others' actions. In any case, both subjective and contextual influences can make a vast difference in how the behaviour of health care's agents and clients facilitates or hinders the implementation of policy and the delivery of care. One of the most sensitive areas is agents' and clients' confidence and morale. For instance, if a promising new drug turns out to have unacceptable side effects over the long run, which require its withdrawal, not only does the health care system suffer replacement costs, many of its agents and clients may lose confidence in drug testing and distribution procedures. This may lead to physicians not prescribing replacement drugs or patients not taking them when they are prescribed. The consequences of having to replace a promising but ultimately unusable drug then are multiplied by the consequences of physicians continuing to prescribe older, less effective drugs, and of some patients' conditions worsening because of not taking prescribed replacement drugs.

At this juncture it will prove useful to clarify much of what we have been saying by drawing a more explicit comparison between health care and law-governed chaotic dynamical systems. To begin with, for the sake of clarity we have rephrased Foucault's descriptions of power relations and ethics by distinguishing among three different sorts of behavioural determinants:

- Institutional influences – the principles, procedures, and disciplines that institutions impose on their agents and clients
- Contextual influences – the behavioural determinants consisting of how others' actions constrain individuals' actions
- Subjective influences – the internal behavioural determinants arising from personal history and individuals' efforts at self-determination

A comparison between health care and a chaotic system like the weather can be put as follows. Institutional influences are comparable to the causal context in which a chaotic system operates. For instance, Earth's gravity, the depth of its atmosphere, and its rotation are causal factors that provide the background or standing conditions in which weather patterns develop. In the case of health care, it is policies, established objectives, and general directives that provide the background or standing conditions in which health care is managed and delivered. Contextual influences are comparable to a chaotic system's particular causal sequences. For instance, local atmospheric pressure, prevailing wind force and direction, and level of humidity are specific causal factors operant in the development of a "high" or a "low" that determines the weather in a particular area. The contextual influences at work in a given hospital, ward, or clinic, and which involve both practitioners and patients, are the local influences on health care management and delivery in a specific location. Just as particular atmospheric conditions determine the weather in any given area, contextual influences determine the character of health care's management and delivery in any given locale.

The foregoing comparison shows how unpredictability in a chaotic system, such as the weather, and in health care, is a function of what we can call global and local causal factors. An area's particular atmospheric pressure and prevailing winds shape and direct the broader, planetary causes of the weather. In like manner, a particular hospital's

or ward's or clinic's contextual influences shape and direct how provincial and federal governments' health care policies and directives
actually are implemented. Local conditions can introduce unpredictability of a high order to the already complex effects of more global
causes, whether it be in weather or health care.

So far, so good, but what needs to be fully appreciated is that the
comparison we are drawing breaks down when we get to subjective
influences. While we can draw suggestive comparisons between
planetary conditions and institutional influences, and between local
conditions and contextual influences, we cannot extend the comparison to subjective influences. There is no comparative parallel in chaotic dynamical systems to how individuals' internal imperatives
affect implemented health care policies and directives. The components of chaotic systems generate unpredictability only in causal
interactions with one another, but health care's agents and clients not
only generate unpredictability in interacting with one another, they
also generate unpredictability in interacting with themselves. Individuals' efforts to be the persons they feel they need to be produce
behaviour that in a physical system would be impossibly random.

To close this chapter, and this theory-oriented section, we reiterate
that the burden of the foregoing, and of the preceding chapters, is
that health care poses unique problems in being inherently unpredictable. When things go wrong with health care, it is not only
because of extrinsic factors like ignorance, error, or disruptive events.
Health care, as a system, has all the unpredictability of law-governed
dynamical systems like the weather, but unlike those systems, which
are law-governed, health care not only has more than enough variables to be unpredictable, but its agents and clients are capable of
independent action. They can act for reasons accessible only to themselves, and they act as they do because of how their reasons are
shaped by the interaction of how they are told to act, how others
around them act, and how they feel they should act to be the persons
they think they are. What most importantly produces unpredictability is the mix of influences. Though responses to particular influences,
such as directives or how peers behave, might be anticipated with a
fair degree of accuracy, it is how people respond to the combination
of institutional, contextual, and subjective influences that is unpredictable. In predicting events in the physical world, say in simple
dynamical systems, we can factor in the degree to which causal influences affect an outcome. We can formulate force vectors and predict

results. As we have seen, such predictions grow increasingly unreliable as system complexity increases. But with people we cannot formulate force vectors; we cannot say that this or that influence will have a greater or lesser effect than another. It is notorious that sometimes people do things for what others see as the most trivial reasons or for reasons that others simply do not understand. Interestingly, when we up the ante by raising stress levels, responsibility, and importance of outcome, we expect people to be *more* predictable because they need to take greater care in doing what they do. Unfortunately, this expectation usually is borne out only in cases where the requirements for what people have to do are quite specific. In more ambiguous situations, contextual and subjective influences seem to dominate, and the result is that we never can be sure just what will eventuate when we set about implementing a policy or directive with a view to maintaining or improving health care.

Plans to reform health care must allow for its intrinsically unpredictable nature. Those plans must take into account our inability to predict the results of changes that might be introduced into the system. More specifically, there is a pressing need to scale back current reliance on top-down control and the framing and implementing of policy on the basis of statistical models and data. As the foregoing chapters attempt to show, macro-level management can be effective only to a point when it deals with large numbers of people, especially when it lacks the enforcement capacity of military or penal authorities. But macro-level management's efficacy is further limited when the people it deals with either bear responsibility for the well-being and lives of others, or are vulnerable and fearful for their own well-being. In those circumstances it is of paramount importance that agents have significant discretion in the application of policies and directives.

This last point brings us to the heart of what application of Foucauldian ideas to health care illuminates. Whether the driving force is genuine concern to provide a nation with the best possible heath care, or is to meet a fundamental social demand at the lowest possible cost, health care cannot be run like a large business. There are just too many variables to control and the bases for projections are too quickly superceded. Most importantly, unlike a corporation's managers, sales staff, and customers, health care's agents and clients interact with one another and, in a Foucauldian sense, interact with themselves in ways that generate inherently unpredictable behaviour.

However, we cannot make further progress at the present level of abstraction. Having established our theoretical base and shown how it applies to health care, we turn now to several key questions. These are: how the present health care crisis arose, how health care reforms have failed, just what entitlements health care serves, and how we might improve things.

PART TWO

The Practice

CHAPTER FIVE

The Origins and Pathology of Crisis

In the preceding four chapters we developed a theoretical framework that we believe can explain the failure of health care reforms to meet their intended goals. In the following eight chapters, we examine the actual management decisions that Ottawa and the provinces have taken over the last twenty years, as they attempted to develop a viable management model for health service delivery. We use our conceptual framework to explain what went wrong with this model. We also review the new round of policy changes currently being considered, as the Medicare crisis escalates. These include the privatization alternative now being actively promoted by the governments of Alberta and Ontario. To ensure a smooth transition from theory to practice, we begin our examination of these initiatives by recalling the two main themes we developed in the preceding chapters.

First, we take from Michel Foucault's work a fundamental insight about human behaviour. This is that there are complex and multilayered influences on people's behaviour in institutional settings, and that these influences are compounded by the normal ways that human actions can be capricious or even random. The result is that predictability breaks down. In effect, it is as if a barrier emerges when systems of human interaction are compounded beyond a certain degree of complexity. This "complexity barrier" has important consequences for the enterprise of managing, because it limits predictive capability to behaviour systems that exhibit less than the critical level of complexity. Moreover, Foucault shows that the factors that contribute to complexity are not just size or scale, but that a variety of psychological factors also play a key role. These factors, which are characteristic of institutional settings in general, reach their highest levels in systems of human interaction like health care, where the emotional loading is intensified. As a consequence, this complexity barrier imposes very definite limits on the design and operation of a functional health management system. This is a reality not sufficiently understood by health planners and reformers.

Second, we draw from our examination of dynamical systems an important distinction between the role of explanatory models versus descriptive or heuristic models in relation to complex chains of events. As a natural system's complexity and variables increase, so does the degree of unpredictability. In the case of highly complex systems, like the weather, the level of unpredictability may reach such an extent that we refer to it as "chaotic." Yet even in these cases it is possible to develop heuristic models that serve a useful purpose in drawing attention to broad trends or illuminating interconnections. What such models cannot do, however, is offer explanatory power sufficient to predict small-scale or local events. A similar distinction exists in the theoretical structure underlying health management and delivery. For health care to be conceptualized at the overall level, which is the task of health planners, the number of variables brought into play becomes immense. At this level, whatever models can be developed must of necessity be heuristic in nature. As we shall see, however, a common belief underlying contemporary health management is that the planning models in circulation are not merely heuristic, but in fact are strong enough to function as blueprints for the actual organization and delivery of localized health services. This is a critical misstep that has played an important part in the failure of health reform to meet its stated goals.

In the present chapter we examine the origins of the medicare crisis. We consider the efforts of successive federal and provincial governments to comprehend the symptoms of crisis, which first arose in the early 1980s and gathered strength in the following two decades. And we preview the different approaches that health planners proposed to bring these symptoms under control and restore an effective management and accountability framework. In conducting this examination, it is important that we clarify the subject matter of our inquiry. It has two essential parts. First, we are concerned with the health care system writ large. The focus of our scrutiny is not on any one individual facility or service such as a hospital or home care program. Our focus is on health care, viewed as an integral whole. It is at this level that planning and funding decisions are made by provincial health ministries and treasury boards around the country, and it is at this level, we argue, that things have gone wrong. Second, we are concerned with the management of that system, where by "management" we mean the process of establishing policies and decisions for the purpose of giving central direction to the system. When governments talk about managing health care, they are not referring to the supervisory processes involved in running a long-term care facility or a community clinic. They are talking about the macro-level decisions that must be made to ensure that the broader goals of health policy and administration are met. These goals have traditionally included objectives such as improving community health standards, introducing new technologies, creating better linkages between the different parts of the health system, and so on. At present, the management goal that occupies most decision makers is the re-establishment of financial sustainability.

Medicare, then, is the operational system by which we receive essential health services. It is widely felt by most Canadians to be one of our most significant accomplishments as a nation. Since the passage of the Medical Care Act in 1966, it has grown from a distant objective to an everyday feature of our lives that we take for granted.

Yet for the last twenty years at least, a succession of crises has beset the delivery of health services. Some of the symptoms of the most recent crisis are evident: backups at emergency rooms, growing waiting lists, delays in treatment, frustrated or burnt-out hospital staff, and so on. For the last several years, these and other surface-level aspects of the crisis have dominated newspaper and TV coverage across the country. One result of the crisis has been significant erosion of public confidence in medicare. In an Angus Reid poll, conducted between February and April 2000, 78 per cent of Canadians indicated they believed the health care system in their province was in crisis, 75 per cent believed the system was underfunded, and 64 per cent believed the quality of care in their province had declined over the last five years. Later that year, Angus Reid reported the emergence of a deeper level of concern: 57 per cent of respondents now believed patients will just have to accept longer waiting times, while 58 per cent feared medicare would be forced to retrench around a scaled-down core of essential services.

This degree of concern is mirrored internally within provincial governments across the country. Ministers of health face stormy sessions with their Treasury Board colleagues, while senior managers in health ministries are becoming outcasts, as their budget proposals consume a progressively larger share of available resources. The Government of Alberta recently replaced virtually the entire team of senior managers at the Department of Health and Wellness, no doubt in the expectation of improved morale and performance.

Faced with this crisis, there is now a developing consensus at both the federal and provincial levels that medicare cannot survive unchanged. Two widely differing and indeed philosophically opposing camps are presently in the process of being formed, with respect to what should be done. One camp, best typified by the Alberta and Ontario governments, believes that no amount of further reform alone can save medicare, and that only by introducing a second tier of privately operated medical services can the gap be filled. The other camp, represented by provinces such as Saskatchewan, Manitoba, and, until recently, British Columbia, believe that new life must be pumped into the reform initiative and that medicare can be saved from within. Some adherents of this view also dispute the real nature of the crisis, and point to what they consider tactics of manipulation by various interested parties, aided by unbalanced media coverage and public gullibility.

Nevertheless it is clear that the symptoms of crisis appear real enough to decision makers, and that consequently we are approaching a crossroads in the future evolution of medicare. In order to better understand the range of public policy choices currently under consideration, we begin with a short summary of events leading up to this point.

When medicare was introduced nationally in 1966, medical science was poised to enter a revolutionary period of innovation and discovery. New imaging and diagnostic techniques, improved anaesthetics, the antibiotic revolution, and an explosion of new pharmacological treatments combined to drive an enormous increase in the success rate of clinical and surgical interventions. In the following two decades, the promise of medicare seemed vindicated, as Canadians in all parts of the country began to enjoy access to high-quality health services and as objective measures of health status such as life expectancy, birth weight, and infant mortality improved. It soon became apparent, however, that this success came with a cost, as health care spending began to exhibit inflationary characteristics quite unlike most other government programs. In the decade 1979 to 1989, total provincial health expenditures in Canada rose from $13.7 billion to $39.3 billion, an increase of 187 per cent.[1]

Initially, provincial governments turned to deficit financing as an expedient. But by the end of the 1980s, the accumulating debt load had become crushing. As deficits reached their peak, approximately fifty cents of every dollar in federal income tax revenues were required just to service the federal debt. At the provincial level, matters became so critical that Saskatchewan was forced to consider defaulting on some part of its debt – an unheard of measure for a Canadian province to contemplate. This aspect of the crisis was averted when Brian Mulroney's Conservative administration quietly provided assistance to Roy Romanow's NDP government.

As deficits mounted, most provinces embarked on across-the-board cost cutting, and many began to reallocate funding internally away from other areas of lower priority, to support growing health care costs. British Columbia, in particular, reflecting the strong commitment to health care of its NDP government in the 1990s, embarked on a program of far-reaching cuts to non-social policy ministries. Between 1995 and 1999, the budgets of social policy ministries, including health, were increased by 15 per cent, while the budgets of the remaining fifteen out of twenty ministries were reduced by 13 per cent. Some ministries, such as Small Business and Tourism, and Environment, Lands and Parks, suffered cuts as high as 40 per cent.

Nevertheless, by the late 1980s, when the deficit run-up was approaching the limits of public tolerance and private capital markets, it became clear that health care could not be subsidized indefinitely by grinding down other government programs: health services themselves would have to be managed. Buttressing this view, health economists brought forward a powerful new argument that carried weight with beleaguered decision makers. This was that if the health status of industrialized populations is considered in terms of gross indicators such as morbidity, mortality, life expectancy, and infant survival rates, there is no evidence that these factors are influenced by relatively marginal alterations in health spending. Canada spends a higher percentage of GDP on health care than countries such as Japan and the UK, but achieves no better outcomes; the United States spends even more, yet suffers measurably worse outcomes. A forty-year study of health spending in Britain between 1951 and 1991 found no relationship between financial inputs to the National Health Service and outcome levels such as hospital survival rates or overall population mortality rates.[2] The study did show, however, that health spending as a percentage of GDP had increased inexorably throughout the period. As the climate of skepticism developed, the view gathered weight that social factors such as income distribution and diet were more reliable contributors to good outcomes in industrialized economies than additional public spending on health services.

The confluence of these two events – fiscal turmoil and skepticism about the benefits of higher spending levels – reshaped the public policy landscape of health care in a profound manner. Moreover, this occurred at a time when public administration in Canada, as elsewhere, was under pressure to adopt more business-like practices. The 1970s and mid-1980s had seen a succession of government initiatives to gain tighter control of spending by the introduction of management concepts piloted in the private sector. Management by objectives, program-based management information systems (PMIS), zero-based budgeting, and a variety of other techniques were all tried in the search for greater efficiency and control. When it became evident that health care delivery must be better managed, it seemed appropriate to adapt a model from the business world. In Canada, as elsewhere, provincial governments accepted the view that only a radical overhaul would suffice to re-establish health services on a more relevant and sustainable level. In the first general attempt to reform health care delivery since medicare was introduced in the 1960s, an aggressive campaign was initiated, directed at almost every aspect of health care management and funding. This reform initiative was based on the incorporation of standard business principles into the management of the health system.

Operational control of the various aspects of health care delivery was amalgamated in new regional health authorities. Vertical management and reporting hierarchies were introduced, replacing informal modes of coordination. Hospital directors became chief executive officers, while head nurses became vice-presidents of patient care. Cheaper forms of treatment, centred on community-based services and home care, were given priority of funding over more expensive acute care remedies. Clinical practice guidelines were introduced to impose uniform approaches to appropriate care by physicians, and attempts were initiated to reform primary care, particularly physician reimbursement practices. Finally, a bewildering array of ad hoc cost-cutting measures was introduced, ranging from administrative fees to delisting of certain procedures or drugs to restrictions in coverage to outright rationing and triage. Because this approach to health care reform was based on standard business practices, we refer to it throughout as the "orthodox" approach. It occupied much of the

1980s and the early 1990s in many Western countries. In chapter 7 we describe in greater detail the Canadian experience with this set of initiatives.

As the results of orthodox reform began to emerge in the mid-1990s, two separate pictures of medicare could be discerned. From a management perspective, it appeared that cost pressures had finally been controlled. From 1992 until 1997, the total provincial health expenditure budget of around $50 billion remained almost flat. For the decade of the nineties as a whole, the total increase was only 21 per cent, dramatically less than the 187 per cent of the preceding decade.[3] Moreover, much of the improvement came in the acute care field, which recorded a spending increase of only 16 per cent, compared to 30 per cent for physicians, 50 per cent for home care and other non-acute services, and 87 per cent for drug costs. A new governance and management structure had also been imposed, based on regional health authorities delivering integrated care. The apparent duplication and fragmentation of the early delivery apparatus, and its myriad of small independent agencies, had largely been swept away. This seemed to promise a more centralized basis upon which to manage health services. Clinical practice guidelines began to take shape, with the promise of curbing wasteful or inappropriate physician behaviour.

From the point of view of care providers and patients, however, many of these operational changes, and a good deal of the political dialogue accompanying them, resulted in widespread confusion about the nature of the commitments that medicare embodies. Instead of clean, clear boundaries demarcating an enshrined entitlement of citizenship, health reforms produced a variegated, convoluted mixture in which fee-for-service procedures existed alongside insured services, in which no coherent logic demarcated service boundaries, and in which local eccentricities obscured the concept of a universal and comprehensive service.

More significantly, the methodology of health reform adopted by the provinces was heavily slanted toward a centralized command and control model, consistent with the analysis that sweeping change was required. Inevitably, meaningful consultation was virtually impossible in these circumstances, both because the new model was almost impenetrably complex and because, from the outset, governments had concluded that coercion would be needed to wrest control from local delivery agencies. As a result, the role of both patients and

providers was fundamentally altered, from knowledgeable partici-
pants to uninformed spectators on the sideline. Many of the difficulties that beset health reform today are a direct result of the alienation
and resentment created by this impositional approach.

A further cause of confusion lay in the fact that even before reform,
medicare was a recent development in Canada, scarcely forty years
old. Its youthful status had prevented a settled currency of civic
dialogue from taking hold. As a result, confusion existed around how
to think about and understand the fundamental concepts of health
care rights and duties. To this day, patients today do not know what
rights or entitlements they enjoy, while caregivers cannot discern the
principles they are enjoined by medicare to preserve. Are our entitlements full-fledged rights of citizenship, the denial of which would
be unconstitutional? Are they instead secured only by government
regulation, subject to change by ministerial fiat? Or are they merely
administrative arrangements, to be shuffled around as requirements
dictate, like a bus schedule?

We might note that the traditional ignorance of medical matters
that the public displays, and that medical practitioners, jealous of
their intellectual property, encourage, has not helped the debate take
a useful shape. The difficulty is heightened by the fact that medicare
is a political commodity and therefore subject to decision making in
an inherently controversial environment. But beyond the inevitable
rancor of political discourse, there is the fact that many decision
makers in the health field find it necessary to cloak the true nature
of their intentions or policies. Even where decisions are purely monetary in nature, the justification provided is more often phrased in
terms of a health rationale. In some provinces, for instance, physicians have lobbied their governments to "delist" a variety of services,
such as wart and mole removal, arguing that these are not medically
necessary services and therefore should not have to be provided on
the medicare fee schedule. Yet those same services may well be offered
by physicians on a private basis, usually at a higher fee. Some people
might feel that if a service is not medically necessary, physicians
should not charge more for it.

We also believe that a major error was committed by the federal
government when it introduced medicare with the Medical Care Act
of 1966 without articulating the civic entitlements implicit in the
statute. This was due to uncertainties about Ottawa's constitutional

authority to specify and impose rights of citizenship in a field dominated by the provinces. Instead, Ottawa has been content to allow the features of entitlement to emerge progressively but piecemeal. Occasionally, when events took an unwonted turn, such as the emergence of extra-billing by some physicians in the early eighties, the federal government has provided additional clarification, as it did with the Canada Health Act in 1984. This attenuated process of defining civic entitlements is deeply rooted in Canada's federal system of government, but it has done medicare no favour.

Nevertheless, if the evolution of public health services had settled at the point attained in the mid-nineties, it might have been possible to declare a truce. Canadians would probably have been willing to accept some of the confusion and coercion imposed by health care reform as the price of sustainability. Unfortunately, as the end of the 1990s approached, it became clear that a pattern of inflationary spending demands reminiscent of the 1980s was re-emerging. After five years of little or no growth, provincial health spending jumped by more than 10 per cent in just two years, from 1997 to 1999. More ominously, these spending increases appeared only to unleash a broader outburst of pent up demands. Across Canada, and indeed in many Western countries, signs of crisis re-emerged. Waiting lists for both elective and urgent procedures grew longer, delays began once more to hamper diagnostic services, and lineups at emergency room locations became common. In hospitals, temporary holding facilities had to be used as wards, while corridors and anterooms were triaged into holding areas. Signs of stress among care providers, particularly nurses, increased, and a significant movement began of trained nursing staff out of full-time and into part-time work, or out of the profession entirely.

More alarmingly, a report on health care costs prepared by the provincial and territorial governments warns that if nothing is done, baseline spending will grow by 244 per cent over the next twenty-five years, compared with forecasted population growth of less than 20 per cent.[4] No allowance has been made for the cost of new technologies or new diseases, factors that have been found to increase baseline forecasts in the past by as much as 100 per cent. The authors acknowledge this deficiency in their model by providing examples of actual acute care usage rates in Ontario. They point out that if standard growth rate models based on population and aging had

been applied to a series of hospital procedures in which new technologies were emerging, predicted levels of usage would have
underestimated actual usage by significant margins.

In 2000, the Conference Board of Canada carried out its own analysis
of health care spending pressures and trends in British Columbia.[5]
The study found that a combination of the rising cost of health care
and British Columbia's aging population will result in public health
expenditures increasing from 32 per cent of revenues in 1989 to 53 per
cent in 2020. The report concludes that this must inevitably lead to
the sacrifice of other government services.

It is this unpalatable prospect which has led the governments of
Alberta and Ontario to conclude that private medicine is now a
necessity. It is this same reality which has prompted defenders of
medicare to advocate yet further centralization and across-the-board
tightening of management regimes. We have therefore arrived at perhaps the most important public policy divide in recent Canadian
history. Perhaps the battle that is about to be fought out over the
future of public health care has overtones of a broader ideological
gulf, visible in a whole range of contemporary issues, from environ-
mental protection to trade liberalization to the future of public education. Certainly it is no accident that the inclination of provinces to
support one or other of the competing visions of health reform
corresponds with their place on the left/right ideological spectrum.

No doubt the origins of the health care crisis also coincide with the
reaching of a high-water mark in government expansionism and the
beginnings of an ebb tide. Perhaps it was inevitable that when public
confidence in the dependability of government began to fade, as it
has done progressively over the last two decades, the heaviest impact
would fall on the flagship program. Yet it seems clear, in retrospect,
that a day of reckoning was bound to arrive sooner or later. The
demands that a universal health system must inevitably make upon
the treasury necessitate the incorporation of an effective management
doctrine and the vigorous maintenance of discipline. Even many
committed defenders of medicare admit that neither of these conditions has been established to date. It might seem, therefore, that there
is at least consensus on the issue of the need for reform, and perhaps
even dramatic reform. Yet, as we will see in the next chapter, there
are still some who either dispute the fact of a crisis in public health
delivery or choose to minimize the issues at stake.

CHAPTER SIX

The Denial of Crisis

Despite the apparent evidence of recurrent crisis over the last two decades, some defenders of medicare argue that the surface level aspects of crisis portray a misleading picture of reality. While conceding the *appearance* of crisis, they insist that nevertheless the *objective realities* of the situation do not bear out the claim that a crisis exists. And indeed, there are points to be made in favour of this view. Given the far-reaching nature of the reform process, it was to be expected that the upheaval would lead to a period of instability. This in turn was bound to fixate the attention of the media, while providing a ready supply of anecdotal evidence for critics to fasten on. Public opinion surveys consistently show a significant gap between what people have heard second-hand is true about the system and what they encounter first-hand. As recently as February 2000, public surveys were reporting that despite their alarm, a majority of Canadians were moderately or very satisfied with their most recent contact with the health system.

Some defenders of medicare also point to the existence of studies that cast doubt on the real nature of some of the alleged features of crisis. For instance, studies of waiting lists have shown that even when waiting times for surgery decline, the public is often convinced that the reverse is true. A recent study reports the experience in Manitoba over a five-year period, during which waiting times for ten common types of surgery, ranging from coronary artery bypass and mastectomy to cataract and hernia repairs, either remained constant or declined slightly. The authors contrast this positive situation with the prevailing view in public opinion that waiting lists had lengthened.[1] It should be noted that despite all the attention to waiting lists, the objective evidence suggests that there is no coherent process in Canada for establishing waiting times. Patients are frequently placed on more than one list, while some physicians routinely add patients to waiting lists as a place-saving device even though no treatment is required at the time. As a result, manipulation of alleged waiting times has become a potent political tactic in the debate over health reform.

The skeptical view of the reality of crisis is best articulated in a recent article by three epidemiologists at the University of Bristol's Department of Social Medicine.[2] They argue that the National Health Service (NHS) is a victim of "the social construction of pessimism," caused by reliance on anecdotal evidence, overattention by the media, and the public's unwillingness to acknowledge that some disease processes are inexorable.[3] Their main point, however, is that where evidence of failure does appear to exist, this is not confirmation of a crisis, but simply an indication that reform efforts must be intensified. Specifically, they assert that the long-standing inability of the NHS to meet demand for a number of high-volume surgical procedures, such as hip replacement and cataract removal, is not the failure it appears to be. Reviewing waiting lists in December 1999, they note that 110,000 people were waiting for day case surgery in England, 21,000 of whom had waited over six months. Yet this cannot be considered evidence of a general problem, the authors write, because "[w]hile in a few parts of the country there are serious shortfalls, in most there are none. If most centres satisfy demand successfully while a few do not, which group is representative: the 10% who account for 35% of the problem or the 10% who have no problem at all?" The solution they offer is to further refine criteria for surgery, introduce better surgical booking systems, and improve throughput in existing facilities. To those who might note that if the solution is that simple, the NHS is apparently drowning in a very shallow pool, the authors remind us of the explanation given for Ophelia's death:

> her garments, heavy with their drink,
> Pull'd the poor wretch from her melodious lay
> To muddy death

We believe that this attempt to deny the reality of crisis while conceding the appearance misses the mark in three respects. First, it seems to rely, at least in part, on a willingness to deflect a certain amount of the objective evidence of failure by a technique of statistical relabelling. In the article referred to above, the experience of a young cancer victim who was denied treatment by the NHS because his prognosis was deemed hopeless is shunted aside as the inevitable outcome of an inexorable disease process, while the suffering of 35 per cent of waiting-list patients is passed over by blaming a small percentage of health authorities for mismanagement. It may be that this form of detachment derives, in part, from the sense that misfortunes become mathematically inevitable if one thinks in broad enough terms. Statistical aggregation certainly has a wonderful ability to camouflage localized disasters. If one attempted to run the nation's health services, or even those of a region, as one large integrated operation, no doubt such a tolerance for failure might commend itself. But as we shall argue below, it is a fallacy to contend that because individual health interventions can be combined statistically to produce an aggregate model, one should attempt to manage them as if they were. We would also note that a minister of health who attempted to discount the suffering of significant numbers of patients or the refusal of care to a young child by this kind of statistical shuffling would soon be looking for a different line of work.

Second, we believe this response entirely misses a deeper aspect of the crisis, which is the turmoil, loss of trust, and deep-seated anger that have accompanied health reform. These are real phenomena, and to the extent they play a part in shaping behaviour, they must compel the attention of decision makers. An elderly person, bombarded with media stories about crisis and expecting to be all but ignored by health care practitioners, may become withdrawn and unwilling to seek help, even when it would have been available. The phenomenon of "cocooning," made visible in the emergence of gated communities, is an illustration of this kind of reaction. Health care providers, believing that resources will not meet demand, may informally or subconsciously ration services even where this was unnecessary. At the decision-making level, the process of health reform becomes so convoluted that it is virtually impossible for decision makers to know what the real facts are. In such a circumstance, the factors that carry the day are the only realities that remain undisputed: frightened voters and angry health care workers.

Third, even if there is room for debate about other features of the crisis, there is no mistaking the seriousness of the financial position. It is quite out of the question that Canadians will permit their governments to return to the near-death experience of deficit financing.

With other necessary program expenditures already being crowded out, there is little more room for internal redirection of funding. And while some provinces may seek additional revenues through minor increases in fees and charges, a general tax increase of the magnitude necessary to sustain demands for health spending is unlikely. Yet the health budget requests now coming before decision makers around the country could only be met, if at all, by a significant increase in taxation. It should be noted, moreover, that so long as health reform results in continued upheaval, the demands for funding will become more vocal, rather than less. Yet an atmosphere of uproar is not conducive to the cool, firm decision making required to stare down these demands. Ironically, it is health reform advocates themselves who, even as they urge the process forward, are often most insistent that governments ignore the resulting signs of crisis. Not Othello, but Henry V, suggests the nature of their exhortation to decision makers:

> Once more into the breach, dear friends, once more;
> Or close the wall up with our English dead!

We believe that this discussion illuminates a fundamental feature of the crisis surrounding health care reform. This is that it is based not just on workplace malfunctions and disorders, but also on a pervasive atmosphere of turmoil and confusion. The evidence of failure is not simply to be found in service disruptions, such as longer waiting times or crowded hospital wards. It is also to be found in the emergence of a systemic confusion in which there is no objective reality. This is precisely the situation that confronts decision makers around the country at this moment. The health care crisis has become the equivalent of a policy black hole, consuming enormous quantities of energy and resources, but admitting of no illumination.

Those who dispute the magnitude of the crisis may be correct when they observe that some aspects of the crisis derive from misinformation, bewilderment, or panic. Their miscalculation lies in failing to see that when these features become preponderant, as they have done, rational decision making is pre-empted. If those factors that obscure knowledge and understanding attain a sufficient critical mass, the crisis becomes self-perpetuating in its own right. Nor is it reasonable to take comfort in the thought that, regrettable though it may be, confusion on this scale was an inevitable concomitant of reform. Some degree of upheaval will certainly accompany any process of change. But when the confusion and disorder that accompany a reform program become disabling, this is an indictment of the program itself.

There is a further dimension to the problem. If, as we will argue in the following chapter, the orthodox model of health delivery has in fact exceeded the complexity barrier, then it becomes impossible for planners and managers on one side of the barrier to predict how the results of their actions will turn out on the other side. It follows that no amount of mere tinkering with operating systems or fine-tuning the workplace will correct the situation. To illustrate the futility of fine-tuning solutions in such a predicament, it may help to consider one such proposal. In a recent and highly regarded study by the US Institute of Medicine's Committee on Quality of Health Care in America,[4] the authors, Linda T. Kohn, Janet M. Corrigan, and Molla S. Donaldson, examine various theses about why things go wrong in the delivery of health care. In part, their conclusion is that the health system is prone to failure because it exhibits qualities they label "complexity" and "tight coupling." These terms are borrowed from a book by Charles Perrow, *Normal Accidents*. "Complexity" is defined by Kohn et al. as follows:

In complex systems, one component of the system can interact with multiple other components, sometimes in unexpected or invisible ways. Although all systems have many parts that interact, the problem arises when one part serves multiple functions because if this part fails, all of the dependent functions fail as well. Complex systems are characterized by specialization and interdependency. Complex systems also tend to have multiple feedback loops, and to receive information indirectly, and because of specialization, there is little chance of substituting or reassigning personnel or other resources.

In contrast to complex systems, linear systems contain interactions that are expected in the usual, familiar production sequence. One component of the system interacts with [the component] immediately preceding it and the component following it in the production process. Linear systems tend to have segregated subsystems, few feedback loops, and easy substitutions [less specialization].[5]

Notice how little effort it would take to translate the foregoing into Foucauldian language about power relations. Multiple interaction is precisely what occurs when the activities of managers occur in a context of constraining behaviour by others, or what we call "contextual influences." Even Perrow's title, *Normal Accidents*, echoes Foucault's concern with accident and inadvertence.

"Coupling" is an engineering term that refers to a system in which two or more components are connected together without cushioning or buffering between them. A system is tightly coupled in which there is strong time dependency between the components, in which the sequence of events is fixed, and in which there may only be one way to reach the goal. Perrow gives as examples of complex, tightly coupled systems nuclear power plants, nuclear weapons handling, and operating an aircraft. Dams and rail transportation are examples of systems that are tightly coupled – events have to happen in the right order and with the correct timing – but are linear rather than complex because of the relatively small number of variables and the predictability of interactions. Universities, conversely, can be considered complex, but not tightly coupled, because although there are a large number of variables, there are fewer interactions between the components and hence greater autonomy in the various parts. Perrow argues that the likelihood of error or system failure will be highest in systems that are both complex and tightly coupled.

Employing this classification, Kohn et al. conclude that the health system is a complex, tightly coupled system. They give as examples medication administration systems, intensive care units, surgical suites, and emergency rooms. All are susceptible to high levels of failure due to the intricacy of procedures, the potential for simultaneous occurrences requiring a correct sequence of responses, and the possibility of distractions. The solutions they explore are essentially engineering solutions:

Complex, tightly coupled systems have to be made more reliable. One of the advantages of having systems is that it is possible to build in more defences against failure. Systems that are more complex, tightly coupled, and are more prone to accidents can reduce the likelihood of accidents by simplifying and standardizing processes, building in redundancy, developing back-up systems, and so forth.[6]

And again:

A critical incident analysis in anaesthesia found that human error was involved in 82% of preventable incidents ... Recommended corrective actions included such things as labelling and packaging strategies to highlight differences among anaesthesiologists in the way they prepare their workspace, training issues for residents, work-rest cycles, how relief and replacement processes could be improved, and equipment improvements (e.g., standardizing equipment in terms of the shape of knobs and the direction in which they turn).[7]

We would make two observations about this line of analysis. First, despite the authors' claim that the focus of their work is the redesign of the American health system, in fact what they draw attention to are individual work-site malfunctions. These occur, or fail to occur, largely unaffected by the broader management issues that confront the health care system as a whole. This is exactly the problem of focusing too narrowly on issues surrounding design or execution, when the real problems are systemic. While Kohn et al. describe their project as building a safer health system, in reality what they are attempting to do is build a safer hospital or ICU. This may be a commendable objective, but it ignores the reality that what ails the health care system viewed globally is not necessarily what ails the individual workplace.

Second, the solutions offered by the authors, which are largely mechanical, engineering systems solutions, will not ultimately succeed if, as we have argued, there are deeper and intrinsic problems that beset health care. It may be that the complexity and tight coupling described by the authors is an inescapable system feature of individual work sites, like hospitals, or more narrowly still, like ICUs. However, these characteristics need not be features of the health delivery system viewed as a whole. Indeed, if complexity and tight coupling are in fact, as the authors argue, a major cause of failure and dysfunction, it should be very much in our interest to design a system free of these features. Rather than start from the premise that these must be regarded as immutable features against which only defensive measures can be taken, we urge a different starting point. This is that complexity and tight coupling, as features of a health system writ large, should themselves be regarded as design flaws, to be avoided like the plague. Indeed, given the vicious circle of unintended consequences and perverse responses that grows up around these features, we would argue that defensive measures are largely useless, and may even make matters worse. The failure of health reform to date is precisely the failure to learn this lesson. It is as if

we were standing downstream watching bodies float past in a river
and pondering a mechanism to snag them, instead of going upstream
to find out why they are falling in.

It is our view that the present crisis over medicare has arisen precisely from treating the delivery of health care on a par with operating a business enterprise, such as a public transit system or a private
utility. We will argue in the next chapter that health services cannot
be administered in this way, because the complex human interactions
involved cannot be productively modelled by applying orthodox
management principles. Health care is different from public transit
precisely because the key variables – the people affected – do not
behave as traditional management theories say they should. In part,
this is due to the special significance that attaches to transactions in
health service delivery. People approach the health care system seeking freedom from pain, recovery of physical and mental function,
and, ultimately, survival. No other service agency deals in these kinds
of heightened consequences on a daily basis. In part, it also has to
do with the heavily institutionalized environment that has evolved
to manage these transactions, and the emotional loading that accom-
panies them. Patients and health professionals take on complex roles
when they enter this environment, and it is the behaviour-modifying
effect of these roles that leads people to respond in unpredictable
ways, or at any rate in ways unforeseen by planners.

As we discussed in our opening chapters, Foucault demonstrates
in *Madness and Civilization* and *Discipline and Punish* how the coercive
and prescriptive regimes of turn-of-the-century psychiatric facilities
and prisons worked to modify the behaviour of those within their
walls. We now know that the same factors are at work in any institutional setting, whether physical like a jail or hospital, or simply
behaviour-limiting, like a probation program or a drug rehabilitation
regime. We also know that the occurrence of these factors is not
confined to institutional settings in which there is a deliberate intent
to modify behaviour. They occur in any environment in which there
is a complex system of human interactions bound together by rules
and procedures. Moreover, we have seen that there is a direct correlation between the degree of interactive complexity of these rules and
procedures, and the production of unexpected behaviour.

As a result, we now know that there is an unavoidable degree of
unpredictability as to outcomes in all complex systems of human
interaction. Indeed, Foucault's views imply that human interactions

are of such a degree of complexity that there is always a residual or underlying element of unknowability about them. At any given time, what each of us does is partly the product of basically random results caused by interactions with others. While we do not share this extreme view, we believe that an important management principle can be derived from Foucault's insight. This is that the predictability of delivery models diminishes as their complexity grows. It is our view that this fundamental limiting factor must be taken into account if we are to address the practical and operational problems surrounding medicare.

The same point can be made in a slightly different way. Over the last twenty years, we have learned a good deal about how individuals' perceptions of their entitlements are in part a function of their self-perceptions, a function of who they take themselves to be. But self-perceptions are not givens: they are malleable and are affected by how people are treated. In particular, self-perceptions are affected by the status individuals are assigned in any complex or heavily regulated environment, such as a health care system. One obvious instance is the ongoing process of "medicalization" that has emerged in recent years. In one of its forms, medicalization involves a process by which various groups in the population come to see commonplace lifespan episodes as symptoms of affliction.

Menopausal women, hyperactive young boys, pregnant women, and elderly people experiencing reduced bone mass have all been subjected to a form of therapeutic reclassification in which their status has been altered from "normal" to "abnormal." This frequently occurs, in the first instance, because normal human processes such as pregnancy or aging may involve various forms of physical discomfort. However, as new drugs are developed that promise to lessen the discomfort, people seek the assistance of a physician to help "fix the problem." Physicians have strictly defined ways of interacting with patients. As a result, a form of dependency arises, in which those "suffering" these conditions move from viewing themselves as part of the normal human condition to thinking of themselves as ill and in need of treatment. The adaptation of medical terminology to describe these new "conditions," and the "treatment" instructions issued by clinicians, further help to define new categories of patients with a new sense of entitlement and legitimization. This emerging sense of entitlement, in turn, alters the self-definition of the individuals involved, and manufactures new clients for the relevant service

organizations. As Jacalyn M. Duffin notes in the preface, the consequence is that delivery of health care is transformed into the business
of managing disease, where the terms "disease" and "health" are
constantly redefined by social and medical developments.

But there is a broader and more ubiquitous form of medicalization,
in which we have grown accustomed to see health care consequences
in virtually all aspects of our lives. From food labels proclaiming the
contents as "cholesterol free" to daily pollen counts to runs for breast
cancer research to the dire warnings that accompany everyday products (a message on a packet of fishing hooks reads "Warning: sharp
objects"), we are inundated with admonitions about possible risks to
our health. Whereas in earlier generations people accepted that they
would eventually get sick and die, now we live our lives trying to
prevent illness. This entails more than just the accommodation of a
new set of priorities in already crowded lifestyles. It also involves
handing over some of our freedom of action and sense of well-being
to the safekeeping of others. This extension of health and illness
concepts throughout our lives has altered both our perceptions of the
health care system and our own self-perceptions. In this malleability
of self-perceptions lies a major source of the unintended, and sometimes perverse, consequences that derail the best-laid schemes of
health planners.

Nevertheless, despite the denial of crisis by some defenders of
medicare, or the preoccupation by others with essentially micro-level
tinkering, governments across Canada are poised to introduce fundamental policy changes. As we noted earlier, two competing views are
currently emerging among decision makers as to how the resurgence
of fiscal crisis should be approached. One camp, represented by
the governments of Saskatchewan, Manitoba, until recently British
Columbia, and to a degree the federal government, believes that
despite the failures of the orthodox approach to date, medicare can
still be saved from within. The primary article of faith among this
group of decision makers is that health services must be available to
all Canadians on equal terms, without regard for income or ability to
pay. Advocates of this position often fortify themselves with the view
that the symptoms of crisis are mainly manufactured and tactical in
nature. The management solution is therefore to stay the course of health
reform while tightening controls and further centralizing authority.

The second camp, represented by the governments of Alberta and
Ontario and most physician groups, believes that the publicly funded

system cannot meet all of the needs that a contemporary health delivery system must satisfy. They look instead to privately funded, privately operated facilities to provide the services that medicare cannot afford to offer. The primary article of faith among this group is that medicare has failed the test of affordability, and that no amount of internal reform will alter this reality. The management solution is therefore to permit the development of a private, second tier of service delivery in a manner that acts as a relief valve for the public system.

We believe that both camps are wrong. If the Alberta/Ontario approach prevails, we believe that important health care entitlements embodied in medicare will be sacrificed. This will occur not by deliberate act or design but, as with much else in health service delivery, as an unintended consequence brought about by failure to understand how caregivers and care receivers will alter their behaviour in response to the new circumstances. If the Saskatchewan/Manitoba/British Columbia approach prevails, we believe that the failures of the last round of health reform will simply be repeated. For beneath the differences in conclusions, both camps approach medicare from the same starting point, which is that health services are amenable to a set of traditional management principles. There is a difference in opinion about who is best qualified to apply these principles – public or private operators – but both believe that what is needed is the firmer application of traditional management doctrines.

In the next chapter we examine the orthodox approach to reform advocated by Saskatchewan, Manitoba, and, until recently, British Columbia.

CHAPTER SEVEN

The Orthodox Approach
to Health Care Reform

In this chapter we examine in greater detail the specific management initiatives that comprise the orthodox approach to health reform. We comment on the shortcomings of these initiatives, and we argue that their failure to achieve the stated goals of health reform can be traced to a fundamental design flaw. This flaw consists of attempting to treat all of the various, and largely separate, components of health care delivery as one organic entity, capable of functioning as a unified system. We argue that there may be heuristic value in visualizing the health system as an integrated whole, in order to highlight potential linkages or identify bottlenecks. But such a model has no ability to function as a blueprint for reorganizing or managing health services. As we noted in chapter 4, the health care system becomes polymorphic if its separate parts are notionally aggregated to form a single entity. That is to say, such a model possesses no predictive powers at the level of detail required to actually direct or manage an operating system, due both to the huge number of variables involved and to the fact that human interactions are not law-governed.

The orthodox approach to managing health care originated in the mid-eighties, when it became clear that publicly operated health services were vulnerable to significant cost pressures well beyond the experience of other public services. Governments across Canada and in several Western countries turned to standard business management principles for a solution. A critique of the various operating features of health care delivery was developed by health planners and policy advisors, along the following lines:

- The various operating divisions, including acute care, long-term care, home care, and primary care, appeared to be poorly connected to one another.
- There appeared to be clear evidence of significant misuse and over-use of resources within each of these operating divisions.
- There seemed to be a disproportionate commitment of resources to administrative overhead, in part caused by proliferation of independent delivery agencies.
- More expensive forms of treatment and intervention were often used when less expensive preventive measures could have been employed.
- There was no reliable database by which the effectiveness of medical interventions could be measured, and by which improved utilization standards could be brought to the attention of care providers and health managers.

In response, health planners advocated a series of traditional management solutions aimed at correcting each of these deficiencies. The following explicit strategies were recommended:

- All of the different forms of health care delivery in a given geographical area or region should be amalgamated to form one large operating entity. It was hoped this would enable greater integration of care to occur while promoting economies of scale.
- Resource priority should be given to home care and preventive strategies, while the prevailing tendency toward more costly acute care should be discouraged.
- Clinical practice guidelines should be imposed on physicians as a means of curtailing inappropriate or unnecessary clinical practices. It was believed that the data-handling capabilities of modern computers made the production of evidence-based guidelines feasible.
- The organization and delivery of primary care should be reformed in order to eliminate perverse remuneration incentives and to better integrate primary care with the rest of the health sector.

We have already observed that the trend toward incorporating business practices in government made it natural to adopt a corporate model when reforming medicare. But there was also another factor at work that played a critical role in defining the path that orthodox health reform would follow. This was that almost all of the leading critics of the existing health management model came from outside the traditional medical establishment. Frequently, they were social policy advisers, health economists, authorities in community health, social workers, or epidemiologists. Most were convinced that the traditional medical model represented too narrow and reactive an approach to the pursuit of public health goals. Many saw the reform program as an opportunity to pursue the broader determinants of health through social programs extending well beyond the boundaries of traditional health services. At the same time, having lived their lives in the shadow of the medical model of health, with physicians dominating the other health professions, they feared that any gains made toward a new model would soon be rolled back once the crisis was over. In effect, they were convinced that it was not enough to advocate merely for a change in health doctrine. They also realized that such a shift in the balance of priorities could only be achieved, and sustained, if a permanent shift in the balance of power between the health professions was accomplished. Hence it came to be argued that the new vision of health services could only be secured within a management and delivery model robust enough to guarantee that the fledgling social services would be given equal status to the more entrenched medical services. In other words, equal status was to be assured by awarding both social and medical services matching positions in an organizational hierarchy capable of according equal treatment and status to both. Without an explicit acknowledgment of the leap thus taken, what had been a heuristic model in the hands of community health experts was converted into an operational doctrine for the reorganization of service delivery.

Taken together, then, the pre-existing inclination to adopt private-sector business practices, along with the emergent critique of the traditional health care model as too narrow, gave birth to a new doctrine of health service delivery. This doctrine advocated converting the various categories of health service into business divisions within a standard corporate management hierarchy. It is a testament to the willingness of governments across the country to keep medicare sustainable that this prescription was dutifully adopted, often at the cost of enormous amounts of policy resources, management effort, and political capital. Across the country, thousands of small

Table 1
Interprovincial Comparison of Benefits Insured by Medicare

	Physiotherapy	Massage therapy	Chiropractic	Naturopathy	Optometry	Podiatry
BC	YES	YES	YES	YES	YES	YES
Alta.	YES	NO	YES	NO	VARIABLE	YES
Sask.	YES	NO	YES	NO	VARIABLE	YES
Man.	NO	NO	YES	NO	VARIABLE	NO
Ont.	YES	NO	YES	NO	YES	YES
Que.	NO	NO	NO	NO	VARIABLE	NO
NS	NO	NO	NO	NO	VARIABLE	NO
Nfld.	NO	NO	NO	NO	NO	NO
NB	NO	NO	NO	NO	NO	NO
PEI	NO	NO	NO	NO	NO	NO

delivery agencies ceased to exist as independent authorities, causing much anger and heartache on the part of community volunteers who had built up these agencies and had fought doggedly, though not always wisely, for their autonomy. Funding priorities were reversed, away from institutional acute care and toward community-based home care and prevention. In the process, a reservoir of resentment was created among institutional care providers that sustains some of the morale problems presently visible in hospitals today. Appropriateness standards for clinical care, long overdue, were introduced. But these proved bitter medicine for many physicians who saw this as further erosion of professional prerogative and autonomy. And, finally, a start was made toward the reform of primary care, a process that is still unfolding at present.

In addition to these explicit strategies, a series of ad hoc changes were also either made or allowed to occur. These included permitting private clinics to provide certain "adjunct" services such as cataract removal, plastic surgery, or treatment of sports injuries; acceptance of "administrative" or "tray" fees for minor procedures conducted in doctors' offices; the practice of delisting certain procedures deemed insufficiently efficacious; and the adoption of widely varying policies in different regions of Canada with respect to adjunct services such as ophthalmology, naturopathy, chiropractic, massage therapy, and physiotherapy. The table one gives a graphic presentation of how balkanized some parts of our health service have become:

It can only be observed that the effect of this piecemeal approach has added greatly to public confusion about the nature of the health care entitlements embodied in medicare. It has also, as we will see, provided a fertile field for litigation and Charter challenges.

It took the best part of a decade to introduce the new model of health care delivery, but an orthodox corporate management hierarchy is today the predominant organizational unit across most of Canada. How then is it performing? As we saw earlier, the promise that fiscal discipline would be restored appears not to have been validated. The new delivery system is already submitting budget demands more unaffordable than its predecessor. More troubling, symptoms of dysfunction are beginning to emerge that appear directly related to the new model. Let us therefore look more closely at each of the main components of this new doctrine.

REGIONALIZATION

When medicare was introduced in the 1960s, the ownership and control of the various health services was widely dispersed. Acute care and continuing care delivery resided mainly in the hands of small community agencies and societies that had historically owned and operated hospitals and homes for the elderly. Religious orders and community service clubs played a significant role. Primary care was mainly based on the family practice model, with reimbursement provided centrally by provincial medical services commissions. In this pre-reform era, the most complex organizational unit was the acute care hospital, and even here decision making was based on a simple model. Through a division of authorities, most clinical decisions were made within the medical staff structure, while administrative matters were handled by the hospital director and his or her (usually his) staff. The interface was informal and based largely on personal contact and face-to-face problem solving.

It came to be believed by health planners that this system was hopelessly fragmented and a source of endless petty rivalries that promoted rather than discouraged barriers between levels of care. Do away with the multitude of agencies, replace them with centralized regional authorities, and at one stroke you gain economies of scale, integrate care, and sweep away administrative duplication and wasteful overhead. To carry out this work, regional health authorities were established by almost all of the provinces (Ontario was the main exception). The standard model was based on existing geographic or local government boundaries, rather than tailored to meet the needs of user groups or service providers. While regional authorities were intended to offer integrated health services on a "whole-of-population" basis, most inherited simply those resources and facilities that happened to be physically located in their territories. Primary care delivery has yet to be included in the mandate of most of these authorities.

Results have been, at best, disappointing. Little evidence has emerged to validate the prediction that economies of scale or improved outcomes would result from integrating health delivery agencies. Indeed, studies in the United States suggest that there may actually be diseconomies.[1]

It is true that economies of scale should be achievable in the so-called "hotel services" provided by hospitals and long-term care facilities such as laundry, food preparation, housekeeping, maintenance, and so on. But at least 75 per cent of the savings in these areas must come through staff layoffs, achievable only by combining small, inefficient operations into larger, off-site production and distribution centres. It was fully intended by health planners that these economies would be pursued aggressively by the new regional boards. But, in fact, few regional health boards have shown either the determination or the sense of empowerment necessary to drive such an agenda against the entrenched opposition of powerful health unions. This failure is one of the major disappointments of the regional model.

Instead, the "corporatization" of health authorities has often led to higher salaries for managers, now titled "chief executive officers," more layers of senior management usually commodicus enough to provide jobs for colleagues displaced in the restructuring, and a paraphernalia of lobbyists, fundraisers, and community liaison officers, all paid to perform tasks previously contributed free by volunteers. Nor have most health authorities recognized the much more sophisticated skill set needed to manage such complex organizations, by recruiting top-notch executives. Regrettably, many regional authorities have become landing grounds for repackaged hospital managers, some of whom were less than scintillating in their previous capacities.

Where previously the fragmentation of services was promoted by petty rivalries between small agencies, it is now sustained by competition between the separate operating divisions of regional authorities grown large enough for such internal dysfunctionality to flourish. Moreover, the walls of these new fortress-like authorities are several times higher than before: a daunting prospect for those in pursuit of reform. The bedlam that a multiplicity of small independent agencies created has been replaced by the inertia characteristic of large, many-layered, multi-site authorities in which the distance between management and care providers has grown dramatically.

In a small community-based facility, it was common for senior managers to know by name most or all of the staff. Difficulties could be resolved informally, before positions became entrenched. A sense of mission and values could readily permeate the workplace. There was close consonance between the professional responsibilities placed on physicians and nurses, and the degree of empowerment vested in them by the organization, leading to high job satisfaction and morale.

By comparison, regional health authorities are bureaucratic, relying on procedure to settle issues, rather than adjustment by interpersonal resolution. Petty behaviour, which would never be tolerated in a small agency, finds room to grow and sap morale. In an environment confounded by all-too-present regulations and all-too-distant decision makers, staff and patients alike grow exasperated. As the author of a government commission on health management in the UK observed, "if Florence Nightingale were carrying her lamp through the corridors of the NHS she would almost certainly be searching for the people in charge."[2]

An example may help to illustrate the self-defeating aspects of overcomplexity. Regional health authorities in several parts of the country have recently complained that they are not receiving sufficient funds to open up new long-term care beds. The result, they allege, is the phenomenon of "bed blocking," whereby patients who belong in chronic care facilities are kept in hospital beds because there are no available chronic care beds to discharge them to. Moreover, this phenomenon of "bed blocking" is frequently described as one of the primary causes of backlogs and lengthening waiting lists in the acute care system. These latter, in turn, are the two most frequently cited symptoms of distress and underfunding in the health system today.

Now bed blocking is due entirely to a systemic breakdown in the internal workings of an integrated health care delivery system. That is to say, it is not caused by externally driven factors such as too many patients or too few resources. It costs between four and five times as much to keep a patient in an acute care bed as it does in a chronic care bed. Therefore, in an integrated system, in which the same organization operates both acute and chronic care facilities, there will actually be a *savings* to the organization if bed blockers in acute care beds are moved into chronic care beds.

Consider the following hypothetical example. A regional health authority operates one hundred chronic care beds, at an annual cost per bed of $50,000, for a total of $5 million. It also operates one hundred acute care beds, at an annual cost of $200,000, for a total of $20 million. Let us assume that ten of the acute care beds are permanently blocked by chronic care patients (many acute care facilities report blockages as high as 30 per cent). Now, if over time, as its chronic care population turns over (a 20 per cent annual turnover is about average), the authority moves its bed blockers into the now vacant beds, and temporarily closes the ten freed-up acute care beds, it saves $2 million on an annual basis. This is enough to open forty new chronic care beds, or to reopen some of the acute care beds, or some combination of the two. In either case, more patients are being treated than before for the same overall cost.

So why does bed blocking continue to occur despite this elementary fact of economics? More particularly, how can it be that bed blocking has become, by common consent, one of the most critical bottlenecks in the whole health system, when the solution is self-financing? The surface-level answer lies in two of the assumptions built into the hypothetical model above. First, as chronic care beds come vacant, hospital bed blockers must be discharged into them. Second, some or all of the acute care beds thus freed up must either be closed, or at least placed off limits to chronic care patients. As we have seen, neither of these management decisions results in less care being provided overall. Indeed, more patients than before can now be treated, a net gain for the system. But in order to make these changes, the organization must be able to exert general, system-wide control over the quite separate admission and discharge priorities of acute care and chronic care practitioners. A regional health board unable to stop bed blocking is, in fact, announcing to the world that it lacks just this ability. Indeed it might well be said that if regional authorities cannot accomplish something as basic, straightforward, and financially rewarding as this, there is no hope that they can pull off the more sophisticated feats they are supposed to engineer.

How could this happen, given that it was to put an end to just such irrationalities that regional authorities were put in place? Narrowly, the answer lies in the dynamics of physician admitting privileges and

referral patterns, which have remained largely unaltered by the introduction of regional decision-making bodies. A physician whose practice contains many elderly patients, and who is accustomed to
placing those who require institutional care in a local facility, may be
quite unmoved by the need to get bed blockers out of hospital beds.
His first loyalty is to his own patients, who, in turn, see the local
long-term care facility as "their" place to go when the time comes.

But looked at more broadly, what emerges is the inability of distant,
regional authorities to recruit the support and involvement of the
many local health care practitioners whose behaviour and patterns of
practice would have to change for the goals of regionalization to be
met. If anything, the goals espoused by such distant bodies become
objects of suspicion on the part of local practitioners. Certainly it
cannot be said that much has been done to win them over, nor is it
clear how this could be done. The benefits of integrated health service
delivery are somewhat abstract compared to the concrete losses in
autonomy and simplicity that regionalization threatens.

Now, it is sometimes argued that there is indeed evidence that
regionalization is meeting some of its goals. For instance, it has been
pointed out that acute care facilities with large operating room throughput can achieve better clinical results in the delivery of some complex
forms of treatment such as open-heart surgery, due to better skill
development in physicians and nursing staff.[3] There is also evidence
to suggest that sophisticated facilities are more likely to utilize the
widest range of technologies.[4] There is also no question that over the
last decade, there have been significant reductions in acute care beds
in Canada. These facts may seem to suggest that regionalization has
accomplished at least some of its objectives. The fact is, however, that
the same results could have been accomplished without implementing
anything as complex or dysfunctional as a regional model of service
delivery. The reduction in acute care beds appears to have occurred
despite regionalization, rather than because of it, driven by the introduction of laparoscopic surgery, better anaesthetics, and expanding
use of out-patient treatment. To the extent that these improvements
are attributable to developments in surgical procedures and patient
care techniques, they mirror similar benefits that accompanied the
development in previous decades of better diagnostic tools or infec-
tion control techniques. That is to say, they came about as a result of
bottom-up clinical advances rather than top-down organizational
restructuring.

Perhaps the most problematic aspect of regionalization is that the values fundamental to high-quality health care – flexibility, compassion, responsiveness, and above all a familiarity with the individual needs of each patient – are those that large bureaucratic institutions are least capable of sustaining. The danger of patients becoming "lost" in such organizations, both figuratively and literally, grows with each additional element of complexity. In Vancouver recently, a teenage boy disappeared under suspicious circumstances. Police and distraught family members conducted a full-scale search of the neighbourhood, until a volunteer happened to check with the hospital. The boy had been admitted twenty-four hours earlier, apparently the victim of a street beating. No connection had apparently been made between a full-scale community search for a missing boy and the unidentified teenage patient in the hospital bed.

We believe the principal flaw in regionalization lies in the imposition of an inappropriate management model. It may be appealing to view the delivery of health services in a city or region as one large, organic enterprise that requires only the overlay of a corporate structure to begin functioning as an integrated operation. This certainly simplifies the work of planners and budget makers. But before an enterprise can take shape, there must be a willing and comprehending acceptance by the staff employed that they are subject to corporate direction, that they work within a chain of command, that their first loyalties are to the enterprise, and that the value of individual actions is measured by the contribution they make to the success of the organization. It must be possible to translate the mission and goals of the organization into specific duties that each member of staff is expected to carry out, and management must have the authority to effectively supervise these duties. And an effective communications system must be feasible, in which staff are kept informed of corporate progress, and through which alterations in direction or procedure can be disseminated. In fact, few if any of these characteristics were to be found in the health care delivery system prior to the introduction of regionalization. Scarcely a single care provider or care recipient thought of themselves either as employees or customers of a corporate enterprise. Patients cannot help seeing themselves and their medical problems as entirely unique and self-identifying, while the primary focal plane and professional loyalty of caregivers is directed to their patients rather than to an organizational unit.

In this regard, a study of government reform in Ontario is of interest. The study, which examined Ontario's experience with the regionalization of local government services, concluded that there were
significant differences in outcomes depending on the kind of service
involved. Specifically, the study found that economies of scale had
been achieved when infrastructure-intensive services were regionalized, such as water and sewage treatment.[5] However, it was found
that economies had not occurred in services dependent mainly on
human resources, such as policing and social services.[6]

In truth, the corporate analogy does serve one useful purpose.
It offers a heuristic device for making the point that fragmentation
of service delivery was counterproductive, and it acts as a reminder
of the benefits from greater coordination. In the same way that meteorological models explain broad weather patterns and climate
changes by reference to the general scientific principles that underlie
them, so the corporate model helps to illustrate the movement of
patients through the health system by drawing attention to factors
that influence the flow. The mistake made by health planners was to
confuse a heuristic model with a management blueprint. In the same
way that meteorological models cannot be applied to the multitude
of small-scale, local weather events, so the corporate model of health
care provides no reliable insight into how the multitude of individual
patient interventions should be managed. This failure to understand
the difference between a heuristic device and a management blueprint is deep-seated in the orthodox approach to health reform.
Advocates of this approach apparently believe that complex goals,
like integrated patient care, can only be met by imposing equally
complex organizational structures. It is as if an airline planner,
frustrated that taxis are not at the airport when his planes arrive,
proposed that the airline company buy up all the taxi firms.

It is our view then that regionalization is flawed in a number of
significant regards. First, it fails conceptually in trying to recast a
largely unconnected series of patient–caregiver interactions as the
integrated work units of a large but homogenized corporate enterprise. Few if any of the characteristics of a corporate enterprise were
present to support such a fiction. More importantly, such a model
collides head-on with the complexity barrier: no system of this size
can offer predictive capability of the kind required by on-the-ground
management. Second, it fails in practical terms by trying to subject
the human interactions uniquely characteristic of health care to

orthodox management principles. There can scarcely have been a less inviting field for the application of such techniques.

We believe that regionalization also failed in another important respect, namely, that one of the key assumptions it made about human motivations is wrong. This assumption was that at the end of the day, the goals of health reform would be sufficiently compelling to command greater support and commitment from health care workers than loyalties owed to existing institutions and practices. We believe this assumption was wrong in two respects. First, it vastly underestimated the degree of loyalty and self-identification that health care delivery organizations create in those who work and practise there. This is particularly true of hospitals. Second, it misjudged the difficulty of trying to preserve a compelling picture of abstract goals in the midst of confusion and turmoil. This latter difficulty was compounded by the very scale of amalgamation: virtually every operating element of health care delivery was to be restructured, most of it simultaneously.

An illustration may be of assistance. Most board members see themselves as proponents and champions of the institutions they govern, and indeed that is one of their primary responsibilities. In a reform environment, however, they may be compelled to become obstacles to the change process, even if they have no wish to be. An example of this occurred in Saskatoon in the early 1990s, when options were being considered about how best to amalgamate health agencies. It was clear that the values most important to the existing hospital boards, such as mission and identity, would inevitably be weakened or undermined in any of the restructuring options then under consideration. To mitigate the loss of autonomy, the boards were told that if they could reconcile themselves to the situation, it would be possible for them to stay on with a reduced mandate. Despite this, board members indicated that they felt themselves compelled to resist the reorganization, even if the alternative were to be the complete demise of their boards.

The most difficult aspect for board members to accept lay in a proposed rationalization of services between the hospitals. Acting independently over the years, the city's three hospitals had developed a triplicate set of core programs in a city that needed only one, or at the most two, of each. It was therefore unavoidable that in any rationalization each facility stood to lose some turf to the other two. This had been apparent to the boards for some time, and each had attempted to reinforce its own position over the years by erecting a formidable bulwark of mission and values around its core services. The result was that when change became unavoidable, the boards were trapped behind their own defensive positions. The chair of one board went so far as to state that if reforms were really intended, the only solution was to "blow us all up, because if we stay on, we won't be able to stop ourselves."

Now, one can take the view that events of this kind are unavoidable in a reform process. Inevitably there will be opponents, and at a certain point they must be pushed aside if they cannot be converted. In the case of board members, who must of necessity take positions that are public and highly visible, there is often no alternative to their dismissal. Yet the same kind of role-adoption that, in this example, trapped board members in an "offside" position, occurs with everyone employed by or associated with the institution. Nurses, doctors, administrative staff, cooks, gardeners, and maintenance workers have gone through the same process of self-identification with the institution and its goals. The more vital and effective the organization, the more closely will its staff identify themselves with its mission. Few if any of these individuals have the luxury of either resigning or provoking their own dismissal, as volunteer board members can perhaps afford to do. The latter can return to their full-time employment and take up other interests. But, for the staff of an organization who rely on it for their income and career, this choice is rarely feasible. Instead, they are left to wrestle with the trap they now find themselves in.

Employees will respond to this kind of situation with feelings of resentment and anger, sentiments that tend to be intensified by the knowledge that all their colleagues feel the same. There is a kind of emotional piling on. There is also a strong personal sense of betrayal, as individuals confront their lack of power to prevent an organization they had come to trust from turning on them. This is a case in point of how contextual and subjective influences can reinforce one another, resulting in behaviour that nullifies the intended purpose of the reforms. It is here, then, that the policy of regionalization is most problematic. For it to succeed, virtually everyone employed in or associated with the delivery of health services must be placed in this situation. How precisely they will channel their resentments, and how they will reorder their goals, cannot be known in advance. How contextual and subjective influences will alter the behaviour of those placed in this situation exemplifies the unpredictability generated by the complex processes of health reform. What we do know is that deep reserves of anger and frustration were created as the merger process was driven forward. If supporters of orthodox reform suspect a hidden agenda in some aspects of the current crisis in medicare, it may not be necessary to look further than the program of regionalization for the answer.

THE SHIFT OF PRIORITIES FROM ACUTE CARE TO COMMUNITY-BASED SERVICES AND THE ADOPTION OF A CONTINUUM OF CARE MODEL

We noted above that the policy of amalgamating health delivery agencies came about because proponents of the orthodox reform approach mistook a heuristic model of the health service for a management blueprint. This led to the creation of a delivery model too complex and layered to function usefully. The same kind of mistake occurred at a different juncture in the reform process, when the issue of a continuum of care was raised. It was pointed out by health planners that if government were to shift funding priorities away from acute and institutional care, and toward community-based care, it should be possible to reverse the tendency of employing the most expensive and scarce resources in the treatment of illness. This policy was supported by evidence showing that clinical treatments were often conducted as in-patient hospital procedures, when they could be conducted on an out-patient basis or in a community clinic. Intravenous treatment of infections, for example, can be safely administered in many cases in the patient's home, yet it was common for patients to spend extended periods in hospital receiving this treatment. And the anticoagulant heparin can be used as an alternative to treatment with warfarin. The latter form of treatment requires patients to be hospitalized under constant observation, while heparin can be taken at home.

A growing body of evidence also supported the view that costly medical interventions could be avoided if an extended range of adjunct programs and services were provided in the community. These services included home support programs, subsidized housing for the elderly or disabled, assisted transport, recreation therapy for people with chronic degenerative diseases, long-term or extended care, palliative care, and hospice services. Most provinces have made heavy investments in these areas over the last ten years. The health ministers note in their report that between 1990 and 1999, spending on extended health services increased by 50 per cent, compared to 16 per cent for hospitals and 30 per cent for physicians.[7] Only drug costs increased more rapidly.

As a result, the notion of a continuum of care was developed to provide a conceptual framework linking these new services to the existing network of health care services. Since this approach was promoted as a less costly alternative to acute care remedies, it has been embraced by provincial governments. Thus Saskatchewan is piloting a new assessment and classification system for long-term care residents titled "Healthy Aging: New Directions for Care," and Alberta has released a policy paper titled "Strategic Directions and Future Actions: Healthy Aging and Continuing Care in Alberta." The notion seems to be that because a group of services, such as home care or subsidized housing, can be located conceptually on a continuum that includes traditional health care services, it is valid to bring them within the policy and funding framework of health care.

We believe this is in fact a further instance of health planners trying to convert a heuristic device into a management plan. It may be helpful, when examining the efficacy of traditional health care services, to consider the epidemiological factors that influence the broader health status of the population. And it may be illuminating, as a reminder about the wider context within which medical interventions occur, to visualize these other factors as a continuum of issues that influence outcomes. But it is another matter entirely to take on responsibility for managing these issues, and moreover, for managing them as part of the health service. Far-reaching consequences come with this approach, consequences that we believe have not been adequately considered.

In addition to the epidemiological considerations that gave rise to the adoption of this model of a care continuum, a powerful unstated objective was also present. This was the distrust of the so-called "medical model" of health care, which was discussed above, and a desire to substitute a social model of health service delivery. Proponents of this shift in priorities were often social workers, psychologists, nurses, and other health professionals with an agenda of their own. While their critique of the medical model, with its alleged overemphasis on costly high-tech interventions had some validity, unstated was their own desire to bring within the realm of publicly funded health services new client groups, a new range of treatments, a new set of methodologies, and a new class of health service providers.

This new model of care has implications both for the financial sustainability of health services generally and also for the conceptual structure of entitlements that revolve around health care. Dealing first with the issue of sustainability, the immediate financial implication is the huge widening of the health care net to accommodate extensive new obligations. When the continuum of care thesis was brought forward by health reformers, it was often argued that this could be accomplished through a shift in priorities, rather than the assumption of new responsibilities. Yet there are strong reasons for anticipating the latter rather than the former. It is often noted that demand for medical services is open-ended, yet for the shift-in-priorities argument to be valid, demand for acute care would have to diminish as new community-based services are extended. There is little evidence that this has happened to date or that it is likely to happen in the future. We must also recognize that the institutional apparatus built up around acute care and the medical model generally, while it may have favoured more expensive interventions, also possessed mechanisms for maintaining a degree of discipline. Perhaps the most obvious are hospital admissions and discharge criteria, which can be developed to a considerable degree of detail. It is much more difficult to visualize effective criteria for admission to some of the new community services, and indeed virtually no work has been done to develop or apply appropriateness standards in this field.

We also must consider the difficulties that arise when two separate policy and funding frameworks are brought together under the same roof. For example, prescription drugs administered to patients in hospital are paid for by the hospital and are not charged to the patient. By comparison, the same drugs prescribed for a patient in the community must be paid for by the patient. The same is true for a variety of medical supplies such as dressings and bandages. It was possible in the past to sustain this form of differential treatment because hospital care was understood to represent a level of complexity and urgency that justified a different policy. However, this inconsistency is now criticized by many advocates of the social model, and some refer to the differential treatment of drug charges as a "drug barrier" to community care. Of course, the two different policy frameworks have coexisted for decades. They became a source of complaints about inconsistency only when community services were brought conceptually within the framework of health services. The cost of levelling up all of the community care funding policies to match the medical model will be significant. Yet we must expect that this is precisely what will happen as a consequence of adopting the continuum thesis.

Turning to the issue of entitlements, it must be noted that many of the new community-based services offer forms of support and attention customarily provided by families and friends. To the extent that traditional coping mechanisms are replaced by an extension of the health care model, we must expect an alteration in the perceptions of entitlement of those affected. Families may come to have a diminished sense of obligation to care for elderly parents, while those eligible to receive these new forms of care will quickly come to see them as a health care entitlement. Moreover, if the normal process of aging is now considered to require a special form of care and treatment, the self-perception of the elderly will be altered in a manner that will likely involve a greater sense of dependency and foreboding. The Saskatchewan-based Health Services and Utilization Research Commission (HSURC) recently conducted a study that bears on this issue. The study examined the efficacy of preventive home care services in helping senior citizens prolong independent lifestyles.[8] Preventive home care services are a form of light home care provided to seniors presently living independently at home, with the objective of forestalling or deferring the need for institutional care at a later stage. After correcting for health status and use of other services, the study found that seniors who received these "preventive" services were actually 50 per cent more likely to lose their independence or die, than those not receiving these services. It was also found that the average *total* health care costs for seniors receiving these services were three times those of non-recipients.

Now recall the title of the Saskatchewan pilot: "Healthy Aging: New Directions for *Care*."[9] The suggestion seems to be that growing old in a healthy manner has become a matter requiring the assistance of professional caregivers. That there are unintended implications of thus medicalizing the aging process is clear from the HSURC report. Yet this is precisely where the continuum of care model leads, if it is interpreted as a model for organizing and delivering care, which is how the orthodox reform movement has interpreted it. Considering how Canada's demography will evolve over the next thirty years, it might have been wiser to leave some room to manoeuvre in managing entitlements in this field. Instead, we now have an extended model of care in which one end is firmly anchored to the entitlements of the health service and the other stretches into far-reaching management of the human condition.

Thus while the adoption of the continuum of care model may have resulted in some substitution of cheaper community-based services for high-cost acute care resources, it seems likely that the creation of new entitlements and new client groups will far outweigh whatever savings may occur. It might have been better to talk about a continuum of life experiences, rather than a continuum of care, for the explanatory value of the continuum model lies in drawing attention to factors other than medical care, which contribute to health status and health outcomes. By demanding a real continuum of care, to correspond to a conceptual point about the social determinants of health, the orthodox reform process repeated the error that led to regionalization.

CLINICAL PRACTICE GUIDELINES

The documentary record of inappropriate clinical interventions is overwhelming. It has been observed that it took medical science until the early part of the twentieth century to be able to offer odds of better than 50 per cent that someone receiving medical treatment would benefit from the experience. It appears that by the latter stages of the same century, the burgeoning incidence of unnecessary treatments by physicians had once more restored the earlier state of affairs. The causes of this situation, however, are more obscure. Physicians often complain that patients put enormous pressure on them to prescribe treatments or order tests for conditions that are either trivial and transient (colds, back pain, "nerves") or for which medication is of little or no use (prescribing antibiotics for flu). The medicalization of normal human processes such as pregnancy, menopause, loss of bone mass with age, hyperactivity in young boys, and so on has greatly extended the field of patient dependency and inappropriate expectations of treatment. It is also well-understood that the growth of litigation arising from alleged malpractice has initiated the practice of "defensive medicine," in which treatment regimes are recast to meet presumed standards of courtroom evidence, rather than patient need and effectiveness.

It is clear, therefore, that a good part of the problem of inappropriate treatments stems from causes that are both complex and deep-seated.

Despite this, the orthodox reform solution has been to take the problem purely at face value. The reasoning seems to be that if there is
evidence to show that physicians are providing unnecessary treatments, then the solution is to collect the evidence and make it available in the form of clinical guidelines. If physicians still do not alter
their patterns of practice, then ways must be found to impose compliance. The result of this reasoning has been that physicians become
identified as the principal culprits, in need of externally imposed discipline. It follows that the development of guidelines cannot be
entrusted to the profession itself, but must be carried out at arm's-
length. Much of this work has been commissioned by HMOs in the US,
or by health insurance companies such as Blue Cross and Blue Shield.

The result of this top-down approach has been to impose upon
physicians clinical practice guidelines that in large part have been
developed externally to the profession. One consequence has been that
practice guidelines are developed in circumstances that must inevitably be viewed with some suspicion by the medical profession. In turn,
this fosters the perception that the values of health managers and
funding agencies are often at odds with those of physicians. There is
also a realization that statistical models based on large aggregate findings have limited predictive value in individual circumstances, yet
the world of clinical practice is precisely the world of individual circumstance. In addition, because of the time lags required to develop
new guidelines, physicians often come into contact with these requirements only after they have completed their professional training. This
adds to the growing inclination of many physicians to view clinical
practice guidelines with considerable skepticism.

A recent study exhaustively tabulated the reasons that physicians
in the United States do not adhere to clinical practice guidelines.[10]
The study cited the following reasons for this behaviour:

- Many physicians reported a lack of awareness of specific guidelines, ranging from a high of 84 per cent for some illness prevention guidelines to a low of 1 per cent for measles immunization
  guidelines. The median level of lack of awareness was 54 per cent.
- Physicians also indicated lack of agreement with many guidelines,
  citing disagreement with the evidence base and belief that the benefits were not worth the patient risk or that the guidelines represented an oversimplified "cookbook" approach. The percentage of

physicians identifying lack of agreement with specific guidelines was as high as 91 per cent (for the American Academy of Pediatrics ribavirin recommendations).

• A number of physicians also identified personal lack of skill or training as a barrier, while many doubted that specific guidelines would result in a meaningful change in patient behaviour. Sixty-five per cent of physicians sampled identified nutrition education guidelines as unlikely to produce meaningful results

Other factors also contribute to the failure of clinical guidelines to achieve their full potential in altering physician behaviour. There is the problem that since physicians see only those patients who make up their practice, they may rely too heavily on the skewed sample of their own experience. And some guidelines aimed at making statistically small changes in the behaviour of large groups, such as anti-smoking counselling, may not appeal to general practitioners, who see only marginal change as a result of their efforts. Yet population health improvements are largely built on small cumulative changes. It should also be noted that the absence of a strong linkage between physician treatment practices and the burden of paying for the cost of these practices, has removed from physician decision making the important criterion of reasonableness or proportionality.

There is a common factor linking all of these causes of inappropriate interventions. This is that the behaviour of physicians is formed in response to a multitude of social pressures and forces that are largely uncontrolled by physicians themselves. Indeed, none of the individuals or groups of individuals involved in these interrelationships would accept that they control the situation. Each plays a role that emerges from the interaction of subjective and contextual influences that it is beyond their reach to alter. The orthodox approach to the problem of inappropriate interventions, ironically, threatens to make the situation worse. Instead of trying to simplify and disentangle a multi-layered situation in which all of the actors feel trapped, it adds several additional layers of its own. Externally imposed guidelines that embody both statistical complexities and a significant element of coercion are more likely, in these circumstances, to create unintended or perverse consequences than to reduce them. At a minimum, this is not an optimal solution. We will discuss in chapter 12 what we believe is a preferable approach.

PRIMARY CARE REFORM

The current model of primary care practice in Canada is one of the principal causes of unintended and counterproductive behaviour in health care delivery. It is based on a combination of the traditional family practice, supplemented in recent years by the development of walk-in clinics and hospital emergency services. At least three distinct criticisms have been levelled at the current model. First, it is often argued that the current remuneration policy pays physicians on a unit-of-service basis. The more patients a physician sees, the more often a return visit is scheduled, and so on, the higher the remuneration paid. This creates a "volume" incentive, in which financial considerations may induce a level of utilization unrelated to strict medical necessity.

The second criticism is that because most primary care providers work as independent operators, they are not linked in an effective way to the rest of the health care system. An instance of this lack of linkage can be seen in GPs who do not follow up when their patient sees a specialist or is discharged from hospital. A less visible, but more problematic illustration arises in the case of chronic conditions that require coordinated treatment by a range of specialists and providers. Certain diseases, such as asthma, some mental illnesses, diabetes, and Alzheimer's disease, can only be treated in an optimal fashion if a team approach is used, in which GPs, medical specialists, dietitians, psychologists, therapists, nurses, and so on are involved. Many patients fail to receive this "missing level of care" because their GPs, who are their principal contacts with the broader health system, are not effectively linked with other providers.

The third criticism is that the primary care system fails to provide efficient 24/7 service, that is, twenty-four-hour service, seven days of the week. Most patients try to see their GP during normal office hours; go to walk-in clinics during extended hours and weekends, or if their GP cannot see them immediately; and show up at the hospital emergency facility after dark. This system is both inconvenient for patients and horrendously inefficient. Most hospitals report that a major cause of ER backup is use of the facility by patients with non-emergency conditions who should see a GP instead. There is also convincing evidence in billing records of double-doctoring – the practice of patients who go to a walk-in clinic then see their own GP immediately after to confirm the diagnosis. In effect, what has evolved is a family-practice model characterized by strong patient – physician relations but inconvenient hours of operation and inadequate linkages to the broader health network.

Most thinking about primary care reform in Canada to date has focused on the first of these problems – the tendency of traditional fee-for-service forms of physician remuneration to induce unnecessary levels of activity. And indeed there is little doubt that both the attitudes and behaviour of physicians can be affected by remuneration. One such response, known as the behavioural offset or volume response, is well documented.

In 1989, the United States Congress ordered fee reductions in Medicare. Subsequently, those services for which the fees were reduced showed an increase in volume: for every 10 per cent by which the fee was reduced, volume rose by 3.7 per cent.[11]

A study of high-income general practitioners in Ontario (defined as those billing over $400,000 per year) showed that while a small number had practice patterns similar to specialists or diagnostic/therapy providers, the great majority (81.3 per cent) billed for services similar to other GPs. They achieved their higher income simply by seeing more patients. On average, this group billed for 2.6 times the volume of patient assessments carried out by other GPs.[12]

A US-based study showed that the lower fee differential for Caesarean births that Medicaid pays compared to private insurance accounted for between 50 per cent and 75 per cent of the lower rate of Caesarean births to Medicaid mothers.[13]

Over a sixteen-year period in Ontario (from 1978 to 1994) the ratio of intermediate to minor procedures billed by Ontario physicians increased tenfold, taking into account changes in population and age characteristics. This "fee code creep" was most prominent in physicians who had smaller practices and among recent graduates, although it was found in some degree across all GP groups.[14]

To reduce or eliminate this volume response, health planners have tended to favour a capitation-based approach. And indeed there is *some* evidence that capitation models can reduce the "volume effect." In a significant study in Kentucky, utilization of health care resources by 37,444 capitated Medicaid patients was compared with 227,242 traditional fee-for-service Medicaid patients. The study found that where primary care physicians in the capitated program had a significant financial incentive to reduce downstream costs such as writing prescriptions or ordering hospital admissions, they did so. The average number of office visits was similar for the two patient groups, but the average number of prescriptions per year (1.9 versus 4.9), the average number of hospital admissions per year (0.11 versus 0.22), and the average number of hospital days per 1,000 patients (461 versus 909) were all significantly lower for the capitated group.[15]

However, there are also several studies in the literature that dispute the finding that capitation reduces the "volume effect." Hutchison et al., writing in the *Canadian Medical Association Journal*, examined the hospitalization rates of patients in the case of physicians who left fee-for-service practices in Ontario and joined capitation programs. They found that while hospitalization rates fell after the physicians joined capitation programs, the decline matched almost exactly the rate of decline in a matched group of fee-for-service physicians who did not change their payment system. The decline was entirely attributable to other factors common across physician practice.[16]

Hurley and Labelle, writing in *Health Economics*, examined the effect of changes in fees paid to physicians for procedures and utilization of these procedures. The study looked at data for eleven procedures in three specialties across a twelve-year period (from 1977 to 1989) in four provinces. The authors report no evidence of a strong, uniform utilization response. They do report evidence of utilization changes in some of the procedures, leading them to conclude that to the degree fee changes affect physician practice patterns, the effect is procedure-specific rather than universal.[17]

As a result, while it seems likely that remuneration policies do play a part in physician practice patterns, it is by no means clear that we can predict with any reliability what the result of changes will be. What we can say with more confidence is that any policy applied to the profession as a whole, in a top-down manner, is likely to fail for reasons we are by now familiar with. Yet this appears to be the direction in which the orthodox reform approach is moving.

To address the isolation of primary practitioners from the rest of the health sector, it has been urged that the employment status of physicians be changed. More specifically, it has been suggested that if physicians became salaried employees of integrated health delivery agencies, the issue of isolation and delinkage could be addressed. This might also offer a solution to the problem of inadequate office hours and the resulting misuse of hospital emergency facilities and walk-in clinics. Such an approach was tried in a number of communities in Saskatchewan in the 1970s, when a community clinic model, employing physicians, nurses, therapists, and other providers, achieved at least some of the goals of a more integrated service model. It was found that physicians spent more time with individual patients, fewer prescriptions were written, and hospital admissions were reduced. Although the model of salaried physicians working in community clinics is widely used in Quebec, which has a different history of health service development, it has not achieved the same popularity in the rest of Canada. Nevertheless, because it offers a conceptually attractive solution to the problem of dislocation, it is often advanced by the orthodox reform movement as a general model of primary care.

We agree that changes in remuneration alter physician behaviour *in certain circumstances*, and that different practice models, such as capitation or salaried employment in a community clinic environment, may be conducive to the goal of integrating primary care with the rest of the health network. But there is a world of difference in the results gained when a group of physicians voluntarily embraces these changes (as happened with the community clinics in Saskatchewan), and what will happen if changes are imposed by an impatient government on the profession as a whole. Yet this is the route preferred by some proponents of the orthodox reform initiative. The argument goes as follows: primary care is currently poorly incentivized and unintegrated with the rest of health care. Capitation and salaried employment have both been observed in some working environments to alter physician attitudes and behaviour. Therefore, if we impose one or other of these models as the standard form of primary care practice, physicians will alter their behaviour in the desired direction.

This line of argument neglects two important considerations. First, the new set of reimbursement mechanisms or workplace arrangements brings to bear complex, novel incentives of its own. A physician working with a capitated patient list, in which the "volume" incentive has been removed, may now be inclined to underserve patients in need or to give preference to routine cases over complex ones. These counterincentives are matched in some capitation schemes by adding complexity to the capitation formula or by introducing a form of surveillance over patient outcomes. But if we have learned anything by now, it is that complexity, surveillance, and coercion are unlikely to produce the results planners hope for.

Second, it is by no means clear that mechanisms like capitation or salaried employment do, in fact, embody the incentives ascribed to them by health planners. What is known from the literature is only that, in certain circumstances, physicians remunerated or employed in certain ways behaved in a certain fashion. The community clinics in Saskatchewan are a good example of the importance of the reservation "in certain circumstances." In the clinics in question, the staff were all hired from practitioners eager to work in such an environment and who were strongly committed to the project. It is unlikely that the model of treatment that emerged was, in fact, meaningfully linked to remuneration policy. It is more likely that the results arose from the desire of this group of practitioners to work in a model of integrated care. Similarly, when we look at the data linking physician practice patterns to remuneration policy, many of which are US-based, we must remember that these results occurred in a health system with significantly different values than the Canadian system. Chief among these is the allocative role played by monetary considerations at all levels of decision making, including clinical decisions. Interestingly, in two of the Canadian studies reported above, the evidence of linkage between remuneration policy and physician behaviour is weak at best. In the chapter 12 we offer some suggestions about how to approach this complex issue.

Nevertheless, a number of provinces are now actively considering moving to some form of capitated model, and pilot projects are already underway in several parts of the country. It has also been suggested that the administration of the new model should be placed in the hands of regional health authorities, thereby completing the amalgamation of health care delivery at the regional level. With primary care managed at the regional level, the quest to integrate all health services in one unified delivery structure will have been accomplished.

We believe this is an unwise course of action. The implementation by fiat of a primary practice model that many physicians strongly oppose can only lead to a further heightening of dysfunction. To delegate its implementation to regional health authorities that have shown little capacity for effective or sensitive management of complex issues, and to do so in advance of problems with the new model being ironed out, can only make matters worse. All of the factors that we have come to associate with unintended consequences and counterproductive behaviour are present to a high degree in such an approach. Indeed, this is virtually a case study of how not to manage change. It will surely be a misfortune if one of the abiding legacies of the health reform movement turns out to be the alienation of the country's primary health care professionals from our national health service. Regrettably, some health reformers seem unabashed at such a prospect. Yet it is difficult to recall any other field where corporate planners have adopted such an antagonistic approach to valued and irreplaceable personnel.

We believe, then, that the adoption of orthodox management practices to "solve" the medicare crisis has been mainly a failure. While some of the stated objectives may have been met, in every case it has been at the price of unforeseen and unintended consequences more damaging than the original problem at hand. Medicare has been balkanized, bureaucratic inertia immovable by any likely management exertion has been created, and care providers have been progressively alienated and cut off from decision making. Patients have been left scrambling, fearful and angry, and the rights of Canadians, hard won over forty years, are in danger of being overturned by decision makers with their backs to the fiscal wall. Worst of all, the fiscal crisis that precipitated these reforms has re-emerged with a vengeance. For these reasons, some decision makers in Canada now believe that a more radical approach to solving medicare's woes is required.

CHAPTER EIGHT

How Medicare Works

It is our claim that health reform has failed because it embodies deep-seated conceptual flaws that undermine the whole enterprise. In the case of the orthodox approach, the flaws reside in an organizational model so complex that an immense field of unintended consequences and perverse behaviour has been opened up, which has defeated the goals of health reform. Many of the chosen methodologies are either inappropriate to the special circumstances of health service delivery or are so opposed by health professionals that they cannot gain acceptance. Worse still, the lack of fiscal discipline that characterized the previous delivery structure remains firmly rooted in the new model.

As a result, some decision makers have begun to question whether, in fact, a public health service can realistically be managed within the limits of public funding. As we will see in chapter 11, this has prompted the suggestion that the health needs of the community can only be met in a sustainable manner by permitting the development of a second, privately operated tier of service delivery. We refer to this model of reform as the privatization approach.

We argue in chapter 11 that in fact the privatization approach is also deeply flawed. In this instance, however, the flaw lies not in the imposition of an unworkably complex new model, but in a failure to understand the workings of the existing model. Privatization is a threat to medicare, not because it does not work, but because those who advocate it do not know how medicare works. We believe this confusion has arisen because the internal dynamics of medicare as a system are not widely understood. We therefore devote the present chapter to an investigation of these dynamics.

Under the terms of the Canada Health Act, health services in Canada must be provided in a manner consistent with five guiding principles: public administration, comprehensiveness, universality, portability, and accessibility. In the Act, these principles are embodied in the form of operational requirements, as follows:

1 The services covered by medicare are all hospital services, physician services, and surgical-dental services that are medically necessary.
2 The level of care guaranteed is that which may be considered "reasonable."
3 Insured services (those services defined in 1 above) shall be provided to all Canadians, and residence requirements in any province exceeding three months are prohibited.
4 The health insurance plans of the provinces must be administered and operated on a non-profit basis.
5 Insured services must be delivered on uniform terms and conditions.
6 Services must be organized and delivered in a way that creates no impediment, direct or indirect, whether through charges or by other means, to the uniformity of delivery and accessibility of these services.

The first two of these operational requirements could be taken to be the service "deliverables." If the Canada Health Act stopped there, it would mandate something equivalent to a mass transit system. The nature of the services to be provided is stipulated and an appropriate level of service delivery is set forth.

But the Canada Health Act goes much further. In the subsequent four requirements, the principles of universality, comprehensiveness, and accessibility are given a specific operational framework. The reasons for this approach are partly historical and partly constitutional. The structure of medicare was first articulated in the 1964 report of the Royal Commission on Health Services, written by Mr. Justice Emmett Hall, and subsequently incorporated in the 1966 Medical Care Act. Justice Hall was aware of the pressures, and opposition, that the introduction of a universal health service would encounter. Experience with earlier attempts in Canada and the United States to introduce limited public health schemes had shown that public systems struggled to survive if forced to compete with private systems in which physicians could earn more for their services. A combination of natural self-interest on the part of individual physicians and organized hostility by physician interest groups usually undermined the public system. Interestingly, this experience contrasts somewhat with the situation in Britain, where it proved possible to erect and sustain a public system in parallel with the pre-existing private system. We discuss below the reasons for these different evolutionary histories. It was Hall's conclusion that a public health system could be introduced in Canada only if Parliament took the necessary steps to impose a mandatory operating framework that could not be subverted.

To understand fully why Parliament acted as it did, it is necessary to consider how the Government of Canada is obliged to proceed when legislating health care entitlements. First, Canada is a federal system, in which regulatory power rests with Ottawa, but delivery of health care rests with the provinces. This constitutional bifurcation of powers presents an obvious difficulty to a federal government intent on creating a universal system of health services. The method chosen by the legal drafters was to embody the goals of medicare in a series of operational requirements that, when fully implemented, would lead to the desired outcome. Parliament did not specifically define this outcome in detailed terms: constitutionally, it could not do so. Instead, it relied on the equivalent of a two-step process to achieve its goals. In the first step, accomplished by the legislation, the operating parameters of medicare were set out. These included the stipulation of public, not-for-profit administration, the stipulation that services must be delivered in a uniform manner, and the provision that entitlements shall be portable between provinces without residence requirements exceeding three months.

In the second step, Parliament relied on health professionals and administrators, working within the statutory parameters, to develop the actual mechanics of a universal health system. Because this second step occurred at one stage removed from Parliament, through the slow accumulation of what we term "medical due process," it has received much less attention than the originating statement of the broad principles of medicare. But, in fact, as we will argue below, it is the functioning of this body of medical due process, brought into being by the principles of medicare, that determines in large part how health services are actually provided, and to whom.

It was the intent of Parliament in choosing this two-step methodology to ensure that the provinces, each working to some degree in isolation, would in fact create a viable national health service. As we said earlier, this bifurcated approach, while constitutionally necessary, has done medicare no favours. It masked the full intent of Parliament at the time, and it has proven a fertile ground for subsequent obfuscation and misdirection. Had Parliament chosen to articulate, in unambiguous terms, a more detailed statement of the rights and entitlements to be secured by medicare, much of the present-day confusion could have been avoided.

The second reason for Parliament adopting the course it took is that health is not a quantifiable "good" in the sense that air quality or water pollution can be quantified. As a result, it was impractical to impose on provincial governments the responsibility for narrowly defined health outcomes, at least as these might apply to the overall workings of their health systems. Health is also an elastic concept: it would be unrealistic to impose open-ended obligations that could never be achieved. The solution, as we have seen, was to prescribe instead a series of procedural requirements, the presence of which would lead, over time, to the essential goals being met.

Third, it is necessary to recognize that we are dealing with a field in which practical limitations are not a theoretical constraining factor, but a real and ever-present challenge for which realistic allowances must be made in the drafting of prescriptive legislation. The solution adopted by Parliament in respect of this difficulty was to establish the benchmark of "reasonableness" as the target at which provinces should aim. As we will see below, this was a choice of language that has led, in the wake of the Charter, to additional entanglements.

As a result, when attempting to examine the question of what precisely are the entitlements embodied in medicare, we are faced with two difficulties. First, because Parliament was forced constitutionally to underarticulate the full nature of its intentions, we are required to fill in this gap for ourselves by interpreting the broad statutory language that was adopted. Second, because Parliament relied on the two-step device of imposing broad operational stipulations as a way of predetermining the subsequent delivery features of medicare, we are required to understand just how these operational stipulations do, in fact, determine how medicare works. It is a regrettable but evident fact that many health-reform advocates, as well as some of medicare's most trenchant critics, have not taken account of this internal dynamic.

The question before us is this: how do the operational requirements that the federal government imposed on medicare influence the way services are actually provided, and who receives them? A helpful analogy can be found in the workings of the legal system, in the way in which criminal law statutes shape our system of justice by determining how the court system actually functions. The foundations of criminal law are built upon a set of basic principles that include the requirements that trials must be conducted on the principle that everyone is equal before the law, that there is to be transparency and fair play at every juncture, that anyone accused of a crime is to be accorded the presumption of innocence, and so on. These basic principles, many of which originated several hundred years ago in English common law, correspond to the stipulations of the Canada Health Act noted above.

In turn, once these basic principles had been embodied in criminal law statutes, a complex body of legal due process evolved to operationalize them. This body of due process was built up over time as judges developed the rules of court required to guide the conduct of trials. Due process requirements include such provisions as rules for the admission or exclusion of physical evidence, procedures for instructing juries, prohibitions on hearsay evidence, and so on. In our system of jurisprudence, the legal rights of citizens are safeguarded not so much by the existence of broad legal principles as by the rigorous application of due process requirements. It has been said that the history of liberty has largely been the history of the observance of procedural safeguards.

In a similar way, the management of our health care system proceeds from a broad base of operational stipulations contained in the Canada Health Act, to the application of a working body of day-to-day medical due process. Analogous to legal due process, these administrative policies translate the broad values and principles of medicare into a reliable and predictable body of practice by health professionals. Such policies have validity because they derive from the guiding principles of the system, and because they have been found over time – like the rules of court – to be effective in securing the goals of the system.

On any occasion when we visit a doctor or are admitted to hospital, we can see some of these elements of due process at work. Examples include the requirement that physicians make their treatment decisions in a manner that is "blind" to the lifestyle or personal circumstances of the patient, policies for gaining informed consent from patients, and requirements for the maintenance of patient confidentiality. Others have to do with maintaining proper physician–patient relations, providing second opinions, and the like.

Perhaps the most important group of due process requirements, however, are those that determine which patients will receive treatment, and why. In Canada, when a patient requires admission to hospital, he or she goes through an assessment process that gauges the degree of urgency of their condition. It can sometimes be difficult for the public to detect the method of selection in this process. In critical situations, the process may be no more than a summary examination by an emergency room physician, followed by immediate admission. At the other extremity, elective surgery is scheduled on the basis of a more relaxed set of criteria, and patients are admitted as circumstances permit. This can lead to extended waiting times, with patients sometimes being "bumped" to allow more urgent cases to be treated. As a result, the presence of due process may not be evident. This has played a part in diminished public support for and confidence in medicare. We will argue in the chapter 12 that public support can in fact be regained precisely by making known, and explaining, such policies.

In fact, the due process around hospital admissions in Canada is principally based on the concept of medical necessity. This concept has been articulated in some areas of treatment to a greater extent than in others, with coronary care perhaps exhibiting the greatest degree of articulation. The following illustration is drawn from a study by the Institute for Clinical Evaluative Sciences (ICES). In this study, the time patients had spent on waiting lists for bypass surgery was compared with their symptoms of acuity. Other patient characteristics, such as age and sex, were also included. Results showed that "median waiting times differed strikingly according to symptom status, ranging from one day for patients requiring intravenous nitroglycerine drips to control unstable angina prior to surgery, to 45 days for those with stable class I-II angina. In the multivariate analysis, with or without normalization of waiting times, the most important determinant of waiting time continued to be symptom status"[1] Neither age nor sex were found to have played a significant role. The study did find that there were variances in waiting times at different hospitals, and that unequal case-load capacity led to patients at some hospitals receiving surgery later than appropriate. In summary, the only significant factors influencing admission to bypass surgery were found to be acuity-based, and there was a direct correlation between degree of acuity and length of time spent on the waiting list.

In a narrow sense, these results were achieved because hospitals in Ontario that perform coronary artery bypass surgery employ queuing criteria developed by a consensus panel of cardiologists and surgeons. It is the application of these criteria that constitutes medical "due process" in these circumstances. But how did it come about that these, and not some other criteria, would be employed? If the answer seems self-evident, we must remember that competing interests exist that could have claimed prior attention. If a patient is well-off, or occupies a position of importance, if a patient is a friend or relative of an attending physician, if a patient presents with an "interesting" as opposed to routine condition, there may be a natural inclination to give priority over medical necessity. So why do criteria based on clinical acuity carry the day?

Some assume that medical science or physician ethics dictate the primacy of these criteria. But while medical knowledge certainly developed the criteria, it cannot take credit for their ascendancy. The answer is that acuity-based criteria are used as the basis for admission because the operational rules that govern medicare debar other considerations. That is to say, when you stipulate that health services must be publicly administered and operated on a not-for-profit basis, and when you prohibit the delivery of services in any way that creates an impediment to uniformity of treatment, you pre-select for an outcome in which only those criteria that are based on medical necessity will gain ascendancy. To see more directly how the operational rules that govern health care determine outcomes, it is instructive to compare the situation in the United States with that of Canada. The following are a sample of findings from studies conducted over the last decade:

- Writing in the *Journal of the American College of Cardiology* in June 1998, Sada et al. report the influence of payer status on 17,600 patients enrolled in the National Registry of Myocardial Infarction, from June 1994 to October 1995.[2] Sada et al. report that angiography was performed on 86 per cent of fee-for-service patients, 80 per cent of

Health Maintenance Organization (HMO) patients, 75 per cent of uninsured patients, and 61 per cent of Medicaid patients. Similar patterns for use of coronary revascularization were found. The authors conclude that payer status plays a role in determining the use and appropriateness of invasive cardiac procedures: they also found that the Medicaid patients in the study suffered a higher in-hospital mortality rate than the other patients.

- Writing in the journal *Annals of Internal Medicine* in February 1991, Weissman et al. report on reasons for delayed treatment in five Massachusetts hospitals.[3] Data from 12,068 patients indicated delay of care was reported in 16 per cent of cases. Reports of delayed care were from 40 per cent to 80 per cent higher among patients who were black, poor, uninsured, or without a regular physician. Among patients who were both poor and uninsured, reported delays in care because of cost were twelve times higher than among other patients.

- Writing in the *Journal of the American Medical Association* in 1991, Hadley, Steinberg, and Feder report a comparison of treatment and outcomes between insured and uninsured patients in a national sample of hospitals.[4] On the basis of data gathered from discharge abstracts in 592,598 patients hospitalized in 1987, the authors found that in thirteen of sixteen age-sex-race cohorts, uninsured patients faced a 44 to 124 per cent higher risk of in-hospital mortality than did insured patients. The uninsured patients were 29 to 75 per cent less likely to undergo each of five high-cost or high-discretion procedures, and 50 per cent less likely to have normal results in biopsy reports in five of seven endoscopic procedures. Resorting to understatement, the authors conclude that insurance status is associated with a broad spectrum of aspects of hospital care.

- Writing in the *American Journal of Managed Care* in 1999, Zimmerman, Mieczjowski, and Raymund examined immunization practices in a random sample of 1,236 family physicians and pediatricians drawn from the American Medical Association's master file of physicians.[5] The study found that 68 per cent of physicians whose primary payer was an HMO used computerized reminders that patient immunizations were due, while only 34 per cent of physicians paid by Medicaid used such a system. Eighty-four per cent of Medicaid physicians required a physical examination before providing immunization, compared to 49 per cent of HMO physicians. The authors conclude: "The primary payment source of a practice appears to influence the use of proactive immunization practices."

- Writing in the *American Journal of Diseases of Children* in 1992, Arnold and Schlenker examined the relationship between childhood immunization and insurance status in 161 Milwaukee-area physicians who administer immunizations routinely.[6] When insurance did not cover immunization, 81.6 per cent of physicians reported that they left the decision of whether to pay for the immunization up to the patient. Physicians reported that approximately half their uninsured patients declined this option. The authors conclude that "[p]hysicians reported that they do not immunize uninsured and underinsured children as frequently as insured children."
- Writing in the *Health Care Financing Review* in 1999, Shih notes that dialysis patients who had secondary insurance coverage received more prescription drugs than Medicare beneficiaries.[7]
- Writing in *Pediatrics* in 1999, Furth et al. examine the association between utilization of two different dialysis therapies and the profit status of the facility.[8] After controlling for all clinical and population factors, they found that children treated at not-for-profit facilities were more than twice as likely to receive peritoneal dialysis than hemodialysis, compared with those treated at for-profit facilities. They conclude that clinical decision making for pediatrics may be influenced by the ownership of the facility at which treatment is provided.
- Writing in *Preventive Medicine* in 2000, Hsia et al. examine the relationship between insurance status and receipt of cancer screening in 55,278 women enrolled in the Women's Health Initiative Observational Study.[9] They report that lacking insurance is strongly associated with failure to receive screening, independent of other factors such as having a family physician, self-perceived health, health characteristics, or chronic health conditions.[10]

What this comparison of the difference between the United States and Canadian health care systems shows is not a difference in clinical competence or surgical aptitudes or differing views about the efficacy of certain forms of treatment. Cardiologists, surgeons, and family physicians in the two countries can be considered, for our purposes, equally well trained and well equipped. All have taken the Hippocratic oath. No suggestion of malpractice arises from the findings reported here. Indeed, if physicians in the two countries were asked to design admissions criteria based solely on acuity, they would arrive at the same standards.

The variations in admission practices and in patient outcomes result instead from the application of a different set of operating stipulations in the American health system. Not only are there no requirements to impose uniformity and accessibility, and to bar impediments such as financial status, but in fact the opposite is true. Ability to pay, either from personal resources or through insurance coverage, is explicitly contemplated both in procedures for admission and in the selection of treatment. Health care delivery in the United States is different from Canada not on account of competence, compassion, or clinical practice: it is different because a quite dissimilar set of operating stipulations make it so.

It should be noted that in fact there is evidence that factors such as social status do play a part in the way people use the health system in Canada. A number of studies have found that people in lower socio-economic cohorts tend to make relatively greater use of primary care services, but relatively less use of specialist services, than do people with higher income levels and higher levels of education.[11] However there is no suggestion that this is related either to unwillingness on the part of physicians to provide treatment or to the affordability of treatment. That is to say, these differences are not the result of admissions criteria or other administrative policies designed to favour people with higher income status. The evidence seems to suggest instead that people with lower incomes or educational levels are less informed users of health (and other) services, and may also be less persistent in seeking follow-up treatment, possibly due to other competing priorities.

The picture of medicare that emerges from this analysis is as follows. At the top we have an overarching set of principles cast in broad, general language, which promote a health system based on universality, accessibility, and comprehensiveness. Then we have a series of operational stipulations that pre-select certain modes of operation such as public, not-for-profit administration, while debarring others such as the provision of care in a non-uniform manner. Finally, we have an extensive body of administrative due process, some of it highly technical, which has evolved to translate principles into practice. It is through the action, and interaction, of these components that the question is answered: how is medical care provided, and who receives it?

In this sense, the dynamics of medicare are much more complex than, say, a mass transit system or a public broadcasting service. And it is this complexity that makes health management, and particularly health care reform, so difficult. We will argue in chapter 11 that the advocates of the privatization approach either do not understand, or have not given due weight to, these dynamics.

CHAPTER NINE

The Right to Health Care: The Legal Context

We argued in the previous chapter that if proposals to introduce a private system of health care delivery are to be fully analyzed and understood, it is necessary first to comprehend how key aspects of the public system work. In this context, we developed the concept of medical due process, and showed how this body of administrative procedures is analogous to due process in the legal field. It is this system of working rules that ensures that whatever high-level entitlements are entrenched in medicare, such as equality and accessibility, are actually translated into the way medicine is practised in the hospital, in the community clinic, or in the family physician's office. The concept of medical due process is important because it reveals how the dynamics of our health care system actually work in determining the way services are delivered, and to whom.

But at another level, this analysis demands that we now answer a more fundamental question: what kind of status attaches to those entitlements, such as equality or accessibility, which the rules of medical due process translate into practice? As important as the latter are, they are only a means to an end. If the entitlements of medicare themselves have only a transient status, as is often the case with government programs, then they present no obstacle to a reform program based on substituting a different set of values. Hence, it is important that we inquire at this point into the specific status of the entitlements that medicare embodies.

We noted in the previous chapter that when medicare was introduced with the Medical Care Act of 1966, Parliament chose not to spell out, in unambiguous terms, the status of the health care entitlements that citizens were to enjoy. As a result of this omission, a significant area of uncertainty was introduced that has clouded the current public policy debate about medicare. A more precise articulation of the status of these entitlements would have removed much of the confusion that presently besets policy making in the health field. More importantly, we believe that some of the options presently under consideration that threaten medicare would not have been advanced if Parliament had been more definitive. The failure of successive federal governments to define and secure for Canadians their right to essential health services is an indictment of the stewardship of the Parliament of Canada.

Nevertheless, despite Parliament's failure to define health care entitlements as specified rights, we believe it is possible to determine what status these entitlements do indeed possess. This can be done both through an examination of the historical circumstances in Canada leading up to the introduction of medicare, and through a study of recent constitutional jurisprudence in the health care field. We will argue in this chapter that the Canada Health Act confers on Canadians entitlements that have attained, both through the originating intentions of Parliament and the evolution of jurisprudence, the status of legal and constitutional rights. It is our view that the entitlement of Canadians to receive health care has evolved, over the last forty years, to a right of citizenship. We provide an assessment of the historical events surrounding the development of medicare in the following chapter.

It is important to note that we say "evolved ... to a right of citizenship." We have serious reservations about invoking the idea that the right to health care is an "inalienable" right, in the sense embodied in the US constitution. We are uncertain about what is added, if anything, by characterizing rights as "natural" or "inalienable." The notion of a right, pre-existing in the state of nature, is elusive at best. In what follows, we choose to make the more modest claim that there are entitlements that evolve to become rights of citizenship through the workings of such civic institutions as government and the courts.

Canadians enjoy two different kinds of citizenship rights. These might be labelled basic freedoms and due process rights, respectively. Basic freedoms are the fundamental rights of citizenship that we have come to associate with pluralistic, democratic society. Most of these freedoms can be cast in either positive or negative terms; one has the freedom to act in a certain manner, but one is also free to abstain from doing so. Examples would include the following:

- Freedom of peaceful assembly
- Freedom of speech
- Freedom to practise religion unimpeded
- Freedom to enter, remain in, and leave the country
- Freedom to vote in a democratic election

Due process rights emerge in a somewhat different manner. Rather than being fundamental entitlements whose role in a democratic society is unchallenged, these fall more into the category of operational requirements that we have found are necessary to give effect to basic freedoms. Many relate to the interaction of citizens with the state, and in particular with those agencies of the state charged with the maintenance of basic freedoms. Examples would include the following:

- The right to be secure against unreasonable search or seizure
- The right not to be arbitrarily detained or imprisoned
- The right to privacy
- The right to equal treatment without discrimination based on race, ethnic origin, colour, religion, gender, age, or disability

Because they delineate fields of complex human interaction, due process rights are sometimes administered by adjudicative bodies such as courts or tribunals. Due process often plays a large part in the administration of these rights, and indeed due process in the field of legal rights is an elaboration of just those rights. It might almost be said that legal rights and due process are one in the same, with due process requirements being simply the fine print, or technical specifications, for the maintenance and assurance of those rights. Certainly it seems appropriate to think of legal rights in terms of a continuum, stretching outward from basic freedoms through an extended body of due process entitlements.

It is not our intention here to present a definitive treatment of the interrelationship of, and demarcation between, basic freedoms and due process rights. Our purpose is simply to draw attention to the consequential relationship between the two. In order to maintain basic civic freedoms over time, we find it necessary to extend some of the same status we accord those originating freedoms, to the due process requirements that have been found essential to give effect to them. By this cause and effect process the more important elements of due process come, over time, to acquire a protected status of their own. Taken together, our basic freedoms and due process rights denote the liberties and entitlements of citizenship. In Canada, some of these entitlements are guaranteed in the Charter of Rights and Freedoms, others by common law, yet others by the accumulation of legal precedent and Parliamentary practice.

What then might it mean to assert that Canadians have rights in the field of health care? To assert that a right exists is to make a claim capable of several different interpretations. Perhaps the weakest form of the claim occurs when the user wishes to signify the desire that a certain state of affairs should come into being, though without the requisite means or authority to ensure that this happens. This use of the term "right" denotes an outcome judged to be just or fitting or even necessary, but one that the proclaimers may be unable to bring about. It was with such an objective in view that Canada signed the constitution of the World Health Organization, which proclaims in the preamble to its charter that

The enjoyment of the highest attainable standard of health is one of the fundamental rights of every human being without distinction of race, religion, political belief, and economic or social condition.[1]

The use of the term "right" in this context implies no entitlement that any citizen of a country could practically claim: it enhances no one's chances of receiving better or more timely treatment. It is simply an assertion that the human condition would be improved if this state of affairs were to come about.

A stronger sense of the term "right" occurs when the proclaimer bases the asserted right on constitutional grounds. Canada's Charter of Rights and Freedoms proclaims:

Every individual is equal before and under the law and has the right to equal protection and equal benefit of the law without discrimination and, in particular, without discrimination based on race, national or ethnic origin, color, religion, sex, age or mental or physical disability.[2]

In this sense of the term "right," there is an expectation that a government bound by constitutional provisions bears an obligation and responsibility for ensuring that certain civic entitlements are protected. Specifically, it might be argued that since the Canada Health Act is part of the legal framework of Canada, the rights of equality proclaimed in the Charter apply to the treatment and due process entitlements laid out in the Canada Health Act.

Perhaps the strongest sense of the concept of a right, short of claimed inalienable rights deriving from nature, exists where there is an unambiguous expectation that a court of law will uphold the proclaimed "right." Such situations exist most commonly in well-litigated fields, such as contract law, where precedent affords a strong basis for predicting outcomes. The situation is less clear in the field of constitutional law, both because of the greater complexity of the issues, and because of the relative novelty of the statutes. The Charter was proclaimed in 1982, while the Canada Health Act became law in 1984. There has not been time yet to amass the body of precedent needed to afford confidence in outcomes. Nevertheless, there has been a series of court cases in Canada in recent years that, we believe, lends significant strength to the view that health care entitlements are indeed rights that the courts will uphold. We summarize below three of the most significant of these judgments.

In a 1999 case argued before the Nova Scotia Court of Appeal (Cameron v. Nova Scotia Attorney General) the plaintiffs held that in being denied access to infertility treatment, their right to "medically necessary" treatment was denied. The Court found that the decision of the government of Nova Scotia to deem fertility treatment "not medically necessary" violated the petitioners' Charter rights under section 15 (1), which states: "Every individual is equal before and under the law and has the right to equal protection and equal benefit of the law without discrimination."

The Court found that the entitlement of all Canadians to equal health care treatment can be interpreted as an equality right within the Charter. On that basis, the Court found that the petitioners' rights had been violated. However, the Court also ruled the government was entitled to argue that section 1 of the Charter allows governments to apply the criterion of "reasonableness" when establishing program limitations. On this basis, the Court declined to order a remedy for the petitioners in this instance.

In a more recent case before the Supreme Court of British Columbia, several families with autistic children argued that in refusing to fund Lovaas treatment for their children, the provincial government had denied them equality of treatment.[3] Lovaas treatment is a form of intensive behaviour therapy that requires one-on-one treatment by a therapist for up to forty hours per week over a two- to three-year period. Costs are between $45,000 and $60,000 per year, per child.

The government argued that the therapy is unproven, that other therapies exist that are less expensive, that treatment provided by non-medical practitioners such as behavioural therapists is not an insured service, and, most importantly, that under section 1 of the Charter, government is entitled to apply the criterion of "reasonableness" when establishing program limitations. Madam Justice Allan rejected the government's arguments, and found that the constitutional rights of the children in question, established under section 15 (1) of the Charter, had indeed been violated.

The Court's reasoning in this case is of interest. As with Cameron v. Nova Scotia, the Court found that the entitlement to equality in the provision of health care, established in the Canada Health Act, is a Charter right. More importantly, the Court rejected the government's claim that behaviour therapy is not an insured service by pointing out that British Columbia insures other services provided by non-physicians. While the Court did not specifically name these services, it is likely that Madam Justice Allan had in mind such programs as massage therapy, physiotherapy, and naturopathy, which are insured services in British Columbia. In effect, the Court's reasoning was that the concept of equality demands equal treatment of services, as well as equality between individuals. That is to say, not only must existing services be provided on an equal basis to all citizens, but the justifications that lead to one form of treatment being provided must be applied equally to ensure that other services of equivalent merit are also provided. The logic that had led the British Columbia government to fund massage therapy, applied evenly, should have led to the funding of behaviour therapy as well.

Significantly, the Court used similar reasoning to dismiss the government's defense of reasonableness. In effect, the Court ruled that if government can afford to fund massage therapy or naturopathy, it can equally well afford to fund behaviour therapy. This finding, which differed from the reasoning adopted by the Nova Scotia Court of Appeal, is significant because the Court rejected the view, sometimes held in government, that reasonableness is a matter for governments and legislatures to determine. The Court quoted Mr. Justice Iacobucci of the Supreme Court of Canada, in a 1999 ruling: "As a general matter, the role of the legislature demands deference from the courts to those types of policy decisions that the legislature is best placed to make. The simple or general claim that the infringement of a right is justified under s. 1 is not such a decision. As Cory J. stated in Vriend, supra, at para. 54, "The notion of judicial deference to legislative choices should not ... be used to completely immunize certain kinds of legislative decisions from Charter scrutiny."[4] Thus it was the view of the British Columbia Supreme Court that Charter scrutiny can be brought to bear on decisions that governments make either to fund or to withhold funding from health care services. In consequence, the Court found for the plaintiffs and ordered the province to come forward with a proposal to provide behaviour therapy for autism as a funded service.

A recent case heard before the Quebec Superior Court goes yet further, giving weight both to the view that health care entitlements are Charter rights, and, indeed, that issues of fundamental justice are involved. In the case in question, two applicants (one of whom, Dr. Jacques Chaoulli, is a physician) brought a suit against the Attorney General of Quebec and the Attorney General of Canada, alleging that provisions of Quebec's Health Insurance Act and Hospital Insurance Act prevented residents in that province from buying private health care insurance. Specifically, the applicants asked the Court to be allowed to obtain a private insurance policy to cover the costs inherent in private health services and hospital services. Counsel for one of the applicants summarized his client's case succinctly, if unwisely: "I am arguing for the right of more affluent people to have access to parallel health services."

The applicants cited three arguments:

1 The two Quebec statutes intrude on federal powers, and are consequently null and void.
2 The prohibition from obtaining a private insurance policy infringes on rights to life, liberty, and security guaranteed in section 7 of the Canadian Charter.
3 The prohibition constitutes cruel and unusual treatment within the meaning of section 12 of the Charter.

The Court rejected all three arguments, and found that the statutes are valid. The reasoning of Madam Justice Ginette Piche is illuminating. While finding that the prohibition on obtaining private insurance is indeed an infringement of private rights, Justice Piche wrote: "The court considers that *if access to the health system is not possible, it is illusory to think that rights to life and security are respected.* The Court feels that the economic barriers created by ss. 15 HIA and 11 HIA are related to the opportunity of access to health care."[5] Further, balancing the infringement of personal rights with the broader public interest in health care, the Court noted, "*Here it (the infringement) is imminent, but the infringement is done in accordance with the principles of fundamental justice and so cannot be regarded as conflicting with s. 7 of the Charter.*" The Court's reasoning was as follows:

The Health Insurance Act and the Hospital Insurance Act are legislation designed to create and maintain a public health system open to all residents of Quebec. They are legislation that seeks to encourage the overall health of all Quebecers without discrimination on the basis of their economic situation. In short, it is a measure by the government intended to promote the well being of its population as a whole.

Clearly, ss. 15 HIA and 11 HIA raise economic barriers against access to private care. However, these are not really measures designed to limit access to care, but measures intended to prevent the creation of a parallel private care system. Underlying these provisions is the fear that the establishing of a private care system would have the effect of diverting a substantial portion of health resources at the expense of the public sector.

The disputed provisions seek to guarantee access to health care that is equal and adequate for all Quebecers. The adoption of ss. 15 HIA and 11 HIA was prompted by considerations of equality and human dignity, and hence it is clear that there is no conflict with the general values expressed by the Canadian Charter or the Quebec Charter of Human Rights and Freedoms.

In closing, let us consider the question of the balance that should exist between individual rights and those of society.

The Quebec public health system does not enjoy unlimited and inexhaustible resources; all the expert witnesses said so. The same might be said for every health system existing in the world. In such circumstances, it is entirely justifiable for a government, having the best interests of its people at heart, to adopt a health policy solution that is designed to favor the largest number of people.

The evidence showed that the right to have recourse to a parallel private health care system, advocated by the applicants, would have *repercussions on the rights of the public as a whole. We cannot act like ostriches. The result of creating a parallel private health care system would be to threaten the integrity, sound operation and viability of the public system.*

Finally, perhaps having in mind the statement by counsel for the applicants that they were seeking the right of more affluent people to make private arrangements, the Court quoted the Supreme Court of Canada, in the case of Edwards Books and Art Ltd: "In interpreting and applying the Charter I believe that the court must be cautious to ensure that it does not simply become an *instrument of better situated individuals to roll back legislation which has as its object the improvement of the condition of less advantaged persons.*"[6]

The Court closed its judgment by recalling the difficulties that the public faced in receiving adequate health care prior to the introduction of medicare, and ended with this warning: "Those who forget history are doomed to repeat it."

It is our view, then, that the entitlement of Canadians to health care is evolving toward the status of a right, originating in sections 7 and 15 of the Charter of Rights and Freedoms. This may indeed already have occurred: certainly there is a clear movement of judicial thinking in that direction, portrayed by the cases referred to above. Further, there is evidence that the courts are beginning to extend Charter protection not only to the basic rights conferred by medicare – equality and accessibility – but also to the administrative arrangements required to protect these rights. In the Quebec case quoted above, Madam Justice Piche upholds statutory provisions designed to prohibit the evolution of a second tier of health services based on private financial transactions. She does so because she accepts the reasoning that such a system would disrupt the functionality of public health care delivery. That is, she extends Charter protections not only to rights, but also to the instrumentalities designed to protect these rights.

As a consequence, we believe it is possible to detect the concretization not only of the basic health care rights of Canadians, but also the emergence of due process requirements that enjoy Charter protection as well. This greatly raises the stakes in any debate over health reform. Unfortunately, it also adds a further element of uncertainty and unpredictability to public policy deliberations, since the possibility of judicial intervention is now real. Moreover, the field for intervention by the courts is potentially very large indeed, given the vague but sweeping language of the Canada Health Act. As we have seen from the Lovaas case, a key element of Madam Justice Allan's reasoning was that since the British Columbia government funded other non-medical therapies, it could not reasonably refuse to fund Lovaas therapy. This is carrying the doctrine of equality a long way, yet there is nothing in the Canada Health Act to prevent such an interpretation.

We draw two conclusions from this analysis. First, whether governments like it or not, Canadian courts are well on the way to enshrining the right to health care in the Charter. In addition, it must be expected that the key instrumentalities of medicare – what we have called the administrative due process of health care delivery – will also enjoy this protection. Second, as the Canada Health Act is presently written, there is a wide field for judicial intervention in whatever policy directions are chosen; one could almost say it is assured. While in the long run this prospect might seem to offer a route leading to eventual certainty as legal precedent is built up, in the near term – meaning at least ten years – a significant source of instability will be introduced. We must expect that stakeholders on all sides – patients, caregivers, interest groups, industry representatives, and so on – will be disinclined to accept any government decisions they dislike until litigation options are exhausted. Assuming that it is in everyone's interest to minimize this potential for uncertainty, we offer some positive suggestions for eliminating the uncertainty in the final chapter.

The Right to Health Care: The Historical Context

In the previous chapter we showed how the recent history of litigation and court judgments in Canada enables us to clarify the status of health care entitlements. Specifically, we argued that the entitlement of Canadians to receive essential health services has evolved over the last forty years to a right of citizenship. It is necessary to seek this sort of clarification, because Parliament did not, for constitutional reasons, adopt unequivocal language when framing the medicare statutes.

We argue in the present chapter, however, that even without the evolution of legal and judicial thinking, it is possible to decipher Parliament's original intent if one examines the events and circumstances surrounding introduction of the Medical Care Act of 1966. We believe that such an examination adds further weight to the view that health care entitlements have the force of civic rights. Accordingly, we undertake such an examination in the present chapter.

It may help to understand the Canadian context within which public health services originated, if we look briefly at how, from similar beginnings, the delivery systems in the United Kingdom and the United States took shape.

DEVELOPMENT OF THE NATIONAL HEALTH SERVICE IN THE UK

The present-day National Health Service (NHS) in Britain was founded on principles laid out by Sir William Beveridge, in his 1942 report *Social Insurance and Allied Services*. Beveridge argued for a comprehensive program of social reforms, including measures aimed at full employment, a wide range of social services, and universal health care. A sense of unspoken values can be glimpsed in the targets that Beveridge lists as the five "giants" standing in the way of social reconstruction: want, disease, ignorance, squalor, and idleness.

Formed in 1948 by the Labour government of Clement Attlee, the NHS was established to offer comprehensive health services to all members of the public, free of charge. Yet, from the outset, Britain tolerated the continuance of private, fee-for-service, medical care. Attlee's objective was not to eliminate private care, but rather to see that the working-class classes had access to care of their own. The development of the NHS proceeded less on the basis of a takeover of private medicine, than on the premise of extending basic medical care to needy groups. It was assisted by a core group of strongly committed physicians who believed passionately in the moral imperative of bringing reasonable access to working-class people.

The strength of this imperative was enhanced by the impoverishing effect on Britain's population and infrastructure of two world wars, an impoverishment that neither Canada nor the United States experienced to the same degree. While the material losses suffered by Britain were spread across all social classes, and were felt in all parts of the country, the impact was most pronounced in the already vulnerable working-class populations of large, industrialized cities like Birmingham, Liverpool, and Glasgow. Here, it served to exacerbate the grim health and living conditions of an already destitute underclass living in these centres. The alarming health status of adult men in these areas had already come to the attention of the authorities when conscription revealed that huge numbers were unable to pass even rudimentary fitness tests. By this almost accidental means, it became apparent that a significant portion of the population in Britain manifested health conditions associated with an absence of the most basic living standards – decent diet, reasonable housing, and access to primary care.

As a result, the introduction of the NHS was strongly associated with correcting a social injustice and bringing a tolerable level of care to people who had previously received very little. Perhaps because of the magnitude of the task, the bar was set low – adequacy was the target aimed for. From its inception, the NHS had the flavour of a poor-man's alternative to private care. Even today, it is widely acknowledged that private care offers the advantages of greater comfort and privacy, and much shorter waiting times for the 13 per cent of Britons who have private medical insurance. Consultations with a specialist in the NHS system are often felt by patients to be hurried and impersonal, in marked contrast with those in the private system: "in an NHS out-patient session the patient listens to the doctor, whereas in a private practice, the consultant listens to the patient."[1]

To understand the objectives of the NHS, one must understand the role of the class-based system still powerfully in place in Britain after the war. When the NHS was introduced in 1946, the role of the private physician, operating on a fee-for-service basis, was already firmly entrenched in the bedrock of British class society. The objective of Attlee's Labour government was not to uproot or drive out this form of practice, but rather to parallel it for the masses of working men and women who could not afford the private model. It would have been no more practical, in the 1940s and 1950s, to eliminate the class system from the practice of medicine, than it would from any of the other aspects of the British establishment. Perhaps for these reasons, but also because of the clear moral imperative to improve the health status of working-class people, opposition by physician groups to the national health scheme in the UK was much less vocal than in the US or Canada.

Britain, then, created a national health service that in many respects paralleled British society in the first half of the twentieth century. The aspirations of working-class people after the war, and of the Labour government that represented them, was not to create one system of health care delivery, and it was not even to create two equal systems. The accustomed willingness, deep down, to tolerate a lower standard by the working classes, and the manifest presumption of a very real superiority by the upper classes, enabled two parallel systems to come into being, each representing the aspirations and expectations of its principal client group. Britain's health care system is inherently unequal, but then so is British society.

DEVELOPMENT OF HEALTH SERVICES IN THE US

Health service delivery proceeded along very different lines in the United States. From the start, many of the originating organizational initiatives were led by government rather than privately. The first drive to standardize and raise the quality of physician training came from a joint project in 1910 of the American Medical Association

(AMA) and the Carnegie Foundation for the Advancement of Teaching. This initiative, which reformed the structure and delivery of physician education, was largely a private undertaking.

At around the same time, the American Association for Labor Legislation, initially with the support of the AMA, began to investigate health insurance as a way of paying for the rising costs of medical care. Draft bills were introduced in fifteen states in 1917. The AMA's own Committee on Social Insurance, set up in 1916, commented favourably on the need for some form of risk pooling as a way of covering the costs of health services. But in a pattern that was to be repeated every twenty years or so throughout the century, no sooner were bills drafted or tabled than organized resistance began. In 1917, the AMA itself changed course, and played a leading role in defeating all fifteen state bills. It was argued that compulsory insurance was "un-American," a precursor to big government, and an intrusion into the privacy of the individual doctor–patient relationship.

Prior to the Depression, a Committee on the Costs of Medical Care, comprising a broad membership from the health professions, social sciences, and the general public, was set up to look into how the rising costs of health care could be met. In its 1932 report, the Committee found, among other things, that half of the lowest-income families surveyed had received no medical, dental, or eye care in the previous twelve months.[2] The Committee also found that medical costs were distributed in a socially inequitable manner, with 4 per cent of families incurring 80 per cent of the costs. The Committee recommended a mild form of jointly funded health care delivery, with both patients and providers participating.

President Franklin Roosevelt welcomed the report, and promised a national health insurance system. At this point, however, an outcry arose once again both in the medical profession and in Congress. It was charged that the Committee's recommendations amounted to a "sovietization" of health delivery. Fiery speeches on the need to retain individualism in the American body politic were made, and the AMA began expelling physicians who had set up joint practices – and actually took court action against members accused of joint practice arrangements. So great was the outcry that President Roosevelt left health reform off the legislative agenda, and the Social Security Act of 1935 was passed without reference to health funding arrangements.

At the end of the Second World War, the issue of health reform was once again made part of the legislative agenda of Congress. At least seven separate bills were brought before the House during the 1950s. Each one was defeated or withdrawn in the face of ferocious opposition by the AMA and allied business groups. This pattern repeated itself throughout the remainder of the century, most recently when President Clinton was forced to withdraw his health reform program in the 1990s.

As a consequence, the delivery system that emerged as the general model of health service in the United States is the private insurance model, in which the costs are borne by the individual. Only in the case of senior citizens are the costs paid for publicly, through Medicare. The poor are forced to rely either on Medicaid or on charity. As we have seen, there are considerable limitations on both the quality and accessibility of this level of care.

As with the NHS in Britain, this model evolved almost intuitively as a reflection of deeper values and principles at the root of American society. These include a tradition of fierce individualism and an abiding distrust of big government. Health care is less a right, than a responsibility, while equality of access to health care is neither a principle of treatment nor an appropriate objective of public policy.

MEDICARE IN CANADA

In some respects, the evolution of health care in Canada mirrored that of the UK and the US in the first two decades of the twentieth century. Most physician care was on a fee-for-service basis. Hospital care was funded on the basis of a combination of fees, subscriptions, and grants, with municipalities often leading the way, as a means of attracting doctors to their communities. Indeed, the hospital at this time was little more than a workshop for doctors.

Yet there were already indications of a different social philosophy. In 1916, the Municipal Doctors' Scheme was introduced in Sarnia, Saskatchewan, through which physicians' fees were paid by the local government. The scheme spread across the rural areas of Saskatchewan and Manitoba.[3] In British Columbia, where municipal districts were often unincorporated or unformed, the provincial government introduced a Medical Care Insurance Act in 1935, although physician opposition killed the initiative.

Perhaps the two key events that led Canada on a different path were the Great Depression, followed in the early 1930s by the Dust Bowl, the latter centred on the Prairies and on Saskatchewan in particular. While Britain and the United States eventually shrugged off the effects of the Depression and resumed their existing paths, many in Canada were profoundly affected by what looked like the failure of capitalism to provide a decent way of life. On the Prairies, in particular, a mood of determination formed to seek a different path. In 1932, the Cooperative Commonwealth Federation (CCF) produced the Regina Manifesto, calling for organized government action to reduce poverty and unemployment and to improve social conditions. The CCF was elected in 1944 on a platform of social reform, with health reform as the central plank. Hospital insurance was introduced in 1946, with British Columbia and Alberta following Saskatchewan's lead later in the decade.

At the federal level, the government of Prime Minister Bennett attempted to introduce an Employment and Social Insurance Act in 1935, but a constitutional challenge stalled passage. Ottawa asked the British Privy Council to amend the BNA Act, and following the requisite change, unemployment insurance was introduced in Canada. However, this uncertainty over the nature of Ottawa's constitutional powers remained a barrier to more immediate action on the health care front. In place of a national health insurance program, which the federal Liberal Party had promised in its 1945 Green Book proposals, National Health grants were adopted as an intermediate way of getting around the issue of division of powers.

In the early 1960s, it became clear that the Saskatchewan government was preparing the next step toward universal health insurance, with a proposal to introduce medical care insurance. The hostility of the medical profession led the Canadian Medical Association (CMA) to ask the federal (Conservative) government of the day to set up a Royal Commission on Health Services. Emmett Hall was selected to chair the commission – an unfortunate choice from the CMA's perspective. Hall's report in 1964 recommended medical care insurance, based on the five principles of comprehensiveness, universality, portability, public administration, and accessibility.

Saskatchewan proceeded to introduce medical care insurance in 1962, after a twenty-three-day doctors' strike was resolved through mediation. And, in 1966, the federal government introduced the Medical Care Act, based on Hall's five principles. Finally, in 1984, Ottawa introduced the Canada Health Act, which removed an ambiguity about physician billing practices and forced the provinces to outlaw extra-billing.

Thus over a forty-year period, a series of cumulative measures by federal and provincial governments built up a framework of services and entitlements in the health sector that ultimately had the effect of entrenching the fundamental principle of equity in Canada's medicare system.

SUMMARY

The history of the evolution of medicare in Canada shows, from the outset, a desire to introduce egalitarian principles into the provision of health services. Unlike the UK, medicare did not come into being as the working man's alternative to an already entrenched elite service. And, unlike the United States, Canadians from the outset saw the provision of health services on the basis of equality and universality as a requisite of civil society. In Canada, the history of the evolution of medicare depicts the emergence, as circumstances enabled it to occur, of an entitlement of citizenship, made possible by medical science and the striving of civil society for equality of treatment in all matters fundamental to the pursuit of life, liberty, and security of the person.

CHAPTER ELEVEN

The Privatization Alternative

We turn now to an analysis of the privatization approach to health reform. While both the Ontario and Alberta governments have recently introduced elements of private medicine, only the latter has, to date, given this policy an explicit statutory base. We therefore direct our attention in this chapter to reform proposed by the Government of Alberta. In the 2000 Spring Session of the Alberta Legislature, the Government of Alberta introduced Bill 11, aimed at allowing private clinics to carry out a range of both insured and non-insured medical/ surgical procedures. Government spokespeople, including Premier Klein, have assured Canadians that they intend no threat to medicare, and the Bill includes several provisions that appear designed to reinforce that assurance.

Supporters of this initiative argue that such measures are necessary to relieve the pressure on medicare, and that there is no threat to the fundamental principles embedded in the Canada Health Act. Opponents argue that private clinics of the sort authorized by the Bill appear designed to introduce a modus operandi fundamentally at odds with medicare. Public opinion is split on the practical issue of whether Bill 11 represents a threat to medicare or not.

It is fundamental to the Government of Alberta's position that Bill 11 will not harm medicare, and that no contravention of the terms of medicare is either intended or will be permitted. While these assurances may be genuine, we believe they do not take into account the far-reaching changes in behaviour that will result from the introduction of a private alternative to medicare. We begin with a summary of the main provisions of Bill 11.

1 Creation of privately owned surgical facilities
   Bill 11 authorizes the creation of what are termed "surgical facilities" by private operators, in which both insured and uninsured
   surgical services may be provided. Where insured services are provided, the Bill states that the patient will not be billed. Where
   uninsured services (defined as those for which no benefit is pay-
   able under the Alberta Health Care Insurance Act) are provided,
   the patient will be billed by the facility.
2 Introduction of a new class of "enhanced" medical goods and
   services
   Bill 11 permits privately owned surgical facilities to offer "enhanced
   medical goods or services," which are defined as goods or services
   that exceed the requirements of generally accepted standards of
   care. Where such services are offered, the patient can be billed by
   the facility and will not be reimbursed by the province.
3 Prohibition of private hospitals
   Bill 11 states that "no person shall operate a private hospital in
   Alberta."[1]
4 Prohibition of queue jumping
   Bill 11 states that "no person shall give or accept any money or
   other valuable consideration for the purpose of giving any person
   priority for the receipt of insured surgical service."[2]

Of these four provisions, which constitute the main part of the Bill,
the first two delineate a new tier of private health care delivery. The
latter are intended to act as safeguards for the existing mechanisms
of medicare, and also to forbid queue jumping, which the public will
not accept. Read together, these provisions seem intended to create
the appearance of opening up a realm of private care outside the field
of services provided by medicare, while preserving the main values
of medicare in the delivery of clinically necessary services. By this
means, Bill 11 seeks to relieve the pressures on medicare by bringing
private resources to bear, albeit initially in the provision of a limited
range of services.

It has been argued by some that, taken at face value, Bill 11 con-
travenes the Canada Health Act. In other words, the creation of a
second tier of private care, in itself, abrogates the stipulations of the
Act that commit to equality of treatment, universality of access, and
public administration. A readily accessible version of this argument

can be found in the legal opinion drafted by Joseph J. Arvay, Q.C., and T. Murray Rankin, Q.C., on behalf of the Canadian Union of Public Employees. Given the trend of judicial decision making described in chapter 8, this may not be an unreasonable argument, although we note that the federal Minister of Health has so far declined to give public support to it.

We believe the more fundamental question is whether it is possible to introduce a second tier of private medical practice, based on a very different system of medical due process from the public system, without significantly altering either the values or the practical working arrangements of medicare. It may be urged that the establishment of a private system, set well apart from the public system and in every way insulated from it, is a reasonable concession to those who seek the freedom to make their own health care arrangements. The question we must consider is whether, knowing what we do about the inter-relatedness of human behaviour, this is a feasible objective. If, despite the best efforts of policy makers, it proves impossible over time to keep the two systems effectively separate, we must also try to anticipate what the consequences will be.

We believe that the issues raised by Bill 11 can be reduced to the following two questions. First, does a mechanism exist through which some of the values, practices, and operating policies of a private system might, over time, alter the attitudes or behaviour of physicians practising in such a system? Second, if the answer to the first question is in the affirmative, does a mechanism exist whereby these changes in attitude and behaviour could, over time, affect the principles of medical due process that sustain the public system?

Beginning with the first of these questions, we note that there is a large body of evidence in the literature that shows that the outlook and behaviour of physicians practising in a private system of care are significantly affected by financial incentives. In the late 1980s and the early 1990s, the United States Congress introduced a series of physician payment reforms in Medicare. These included the Omnibus Budget Reconciliation Act of 1989, the introduction of the Medicare Fee Schedule (MFS) of 1992, and the implementation of the Resource-Based Relative Value Scale (RBRVS), also in 1992, for pricing physician services. The intent of these various measures ranged from trying to encourage the substitution of cheaper interventions to redistributing remuneration between specialties to across-the-board budget cutting. The magnitude of these changes provides a broad base of data for examining how physicians in a private system of care respond to payment mechanisms. While the sheer complexity of the changes makes analysis difficult, as does the repeated tinkering that Congress engaged in, a number of general trends are nevertheless evident in the data.

First, as relative fee schedules were altered to favour one form of procedure over another, physicians tended to substitute the procedure that maximized their incomes, as the following study showed. When the RBRVS was introduced, one of its objectives was to induce physicians to substitute a less costly form of coronary care, percutaneous transluminal coronary artery (PCTA) treatment, for a more expensive form of treatment, coronary artery bypass graft (CABG) surgery. Okunade and Miles examined the effect of this aspect of the RBRVS on physician practice patterns. They found that when the fee was increased for PCTA treatment and decreased for CABG surgery, utilization of the former increased while the latter decreased. There were no clinical or population-based reasons to account for this shift in practice.[3]

A second trend that can be found in these, and other US data, is the tendency of physicians to favour treating patients whose insurance status offers a higher level of reimbursement, as the following examples show. Lee and Gillis examined the impact of the Medicare fee reforms on physician willingness to treat new Medicare patients. They found that while there was little change in the number of visits provided to existing Medicare patients, fewer physicians were willing to accept all new Medicare patients. The number of physicians who refused to accept any new Medicare patients also grew.[4]

Zhang examined physicians' decisions about participation in Medicare in relation to reimbursement policy. The study showed that when Medicare reimbursement policy is less generous than private insurance rates, the participation of physicians in Medicare is negatively affected.[5]

Haber and Mitchell examined the question of whether MFS changes in physician reimbursement affected access to care for vulnerable Medicare patients. They found that there were "substantial utilization gaps between vulnerable and non-vulnerable sub-populations for primary care services, as well as for high-cost procedures during episodes of care for acute myocardial infarctions."[6]

Several studies reported variations in levels of obstetric care received by women who were either Medicaid patients or who were uninsured. Onion et al. studied the variation in Caesarean section rates between insured, Medicaid, and uninsured patients in New England between 1990 and 1992. They found that "[a]ge-adjusted cesarean section rates for insured women (15.71%) were significantly higher than those for Medicaid (14.35%) and uninsured (12.85%) women." They also noted that the differences found in New England are much lower than those reported elsewhere in the United States.[7]

Rice et al. examined how the volume of privately insured services provided in hospital in-patient and out-patient departments changes in response to reductions in Medicare fee levels relative to private rates. They used data from seventeen major procedure groups, spanning 182 hospitals, covering a period of twenty-four months before Medicare surgical fees were reduced to twenty-one months after the reduction (1988 to 1991). They found that for a number of procedure groups, though not in all, physicians reacted to the relative fee reduction by treating fewer Medicare patients.[8]

A study in Northern California reported that physicians limited the number of Medicaid obstetric patients they were willing to treat because of administrative inconvenience and insufficient reimbursement.[9]

It is apparent, then, that the operation of financial incentives in a private system of care represents a mechanism that can alter physician practice and attitudes. If the findings noted above are combined with those in chapter 8, dealing with the difference between practice patterns in Canada and the United States, it becomes apparent that physician behaviour can indeed be affected by the operating policies and values of a private system of practice. The answer to our first question is therefore in the affirmative. There do appear to be mechanisms whereby the operating policies of private systems of care can influence the behaviour of physicians practising within them. We would note that this is scarcely a surprising discovery. Human behaviour is subject to many influences, financial considerations certainly among them. What is perhaps more surprising is the reluctance of advocates for private medicine to take this factor into account. It is one of the more discouraging truths about public administration that unintended consequences are frequently wished away, even when they are visible to the naked eye. If crisis concentrates the mind, it seems also to offer an excuse for ignoring unpalatable truths.

We move then to our second question: is it plausible that these alterations in physician attitudes and practice could lead to changes in medical due process within the public system? In what follows, we detail seven mechanisms whereby such changes could occur.

1 Recategorization

If a patient comes to a private surgical clinic for treatment, the attending physician must first determine if the treatment is insured or not. If it is, no additional charge will be levied and medicare will pay for the treatment. If it is not, the clinic may charge whatever the market will bear. This might seem straightforward, but in fact it is not. There are already, within existing standards of care, unavoidable degrees of ambiguity. An adolescent girl presents with a disfiguring but not disabling condition. Is this insurable or not? Most physicians presented with this judgment call in our public system of care would be motivated to find the condition insurable, thereby making treatment feasible for the patient The interests of the physician and patient coincide, enabling the physician to act as the patient's advocate, a role consonant with physician ethics.

A physician practising within a private surgical clinic, however, faces a different configuration of interests. It is now very much in his or her financial interest to find the treatment uninsurable, thereby increasing the level of remuneration considerably. Simply by recategorizing the condition, therefore, a different concept of due process can be validated. The role of advocate is no longer viable in this situation, bringing the physician into conflict with a basic value set of the profession. In fact, this basic dilemma takes several shapes. Consider a physician whose practice includes both public and private patients. He or she has a clear financial incentive to devote more time to private patients, and indeed, as we have seen, there is evidence of this behaviour in the US literature. Such a physician also has obligations to his or her partners, if the enterprise is a joint one, as such practices often are. Colleagues in the clinic, who may be anaesthesiologists, radiologists, or nursing staff can maintain their income only if the admitting physician brings in enough business to go around.

It is not our purpose to suggest that an inherent conflict exists between the interests of physicians and those of patients. A recent US study demonstrated that physicians frequently manipulate rules to benefit their patients. Wynia et al. surveyed 1,124 physicians in a national random sample in 1998 to determine the frequency with which physicians manipulated reimbursement rules to benefit their patients.[10] The authors reported that 39 per cent of respondents had used at least one of the following tactics in the preceding year: exaggerating the severity of patients' conditions; changing patients' billing diagnoses; and reporting signs or symptoms that patients did not have to help the patients secure coverage for needed care. Our point is simply that physician behaviour is subject to manipulation or alteration based on the configuration of interests that physicians perceive in a given situation. In the study reported here, the interests that physicians found compelling were those of their patients. But this points to a deeper significance than supporters of privatization may acknowledge, in the way basic concepts of medical due process can be altered by reforms of the health system.

2 Service enhancement

Bill 11 permits the introduction of a new class of "enhanced" medical goods and services. These are services that go beyond the requirements of current standards of care. In effect, any treatment that exceeds a minimally acceptable level of care can be deemed "uninsured" for the purposes of private surgical facilities. It is not difficult to envisage behavioural implications in this provision. Consider the following three hypothetical case studies.

Case 1: A seventy-five-year-old woman presents with early-stage cataract. Current standards of care suggest she should have lens replacement in six months, in which case medicare will pay the cost. She is told that she can have the treatment immediately, but only if she is willing to have the treatment carried out privately. This is apparently sanctioned by Bill 11, because the service can be deemed "enhanced" beyond current standards of care, in virtue of the treatment being carried out earlier than medically necessary. Note that there may be no medical benefit associated with such an accelerated treatment; there may even be a small but measurable risk, since even the most routine surgical procedures can go amiss.

Case 2: An eighty-year-old man presents with arthritis of the hip. Contemporary standards of care suggest hip replacement, using a regular stainless steel ball joint. Current waiting lists suggest a waiting time of about four months. He is told that he can have the operation immediately, using an "enhanced" alloy ball joint, if he is willing to have the procedure carried out privately. This is apparently feasible under Bill 11, because the medical goods to be used are of a higher quality than is medically necessary.

Case 3: A forty-year-old man presents with chronic knee pain resulting from a sports injury. Contemporary standards of care suggest replacement with a prosthetic knee joint. Current waiting lists suggest a six-month waiting time. He is told that he can have the operation immediately, with the procedure costs of $1,500 paid for by medicare. However, it will be necessary for him, or a member of his family, to purchase other, non-insured services from the clinic, in the amount of $2,000. He is given a list of available services to choose from, which may include various cosmetic procedures, such as skin treatments or hair removal. Since these services are not medically necessary, and quite possibly of dubious value in any other sense, their main function is to serve as the basis for a "cover charge." This is apparently feasible under Bill 11, because the payment charged is, at least nominally, not for an insured service. It is believed that such transactions may be occurring in some private clinics in British Columbia at the present time.

In all of these cases, there is a significant monetary interest to the attending physician in providing a treatment in excess of current standards of care. This interest is in opposition to the monetary interests of the patient. It may reasonably be expected that behaviour changes on the part of both physicians and patients will ensue, in response to these visible alterations in their interests.

3 Patient reassignment

We cannot expect that alterations of physician behaviour will be confined to practice within a private clinic. Most physicians, and virtually all specialists, have admitting privileges at hospitals in their area. Here also, they will face a conflict of interest not previously present. Any patient they treat in hospital, rather than privately at their surgical facility, represents lost revenue. Over time, this may reasonably be expected to result in behavioural shifts, as patients who could, and should, have been treated in the public system are reassigned by their physicians to the private system. We note that one partial solution to this foreseeable problem, namely, requiring physicians employed at private clinics to surrender privileges at public facilities and opt out of medicare, was not adopted in Bill 11. We must therefore anticipate seepage of altered perceptions and interests from their originating point in private clinics into the broader public system as physicians tend irons in both fires.

4 Labour withdrawal

We must also anticipate changes in the utilization, and management, of hospitals in the public system if physicians share their time between several facilities. A recent study in Norway suggests that waiting times at public hospitals may increase if physicians with admitting privileges are also allowed to work in private practice in their spare time.[11] This occurs because as physicians withdraw their services to practice part-time in private facilities, the relative inelasticity of demand for health care ensures that more patients come forward to replace those who seek private care. But, of course, there are now fewer physician resources available to the public system as a result of the transfer of some physicians to private facilities.

Nor is this problem confined narrowly to a reduction in service levels associated with the withdrawal of labour. It also appears that physicians who practise at several facilities tend to impose a greater burden on the resources of those facilities, as they attempt to compensate for their reduced availability. A us-based study examined the utilization of hospital resources among physicians who were affiliated with more than one hospital. The study was based on 1991 data from the Medicare National Claims History File, and focused on 33,756 physicians in seven states. Those who were affiliated with only one hospital had resource-use profiles 2.1 per cent below the sample mean, those with affiliations at two sites had profiles 2.3 per cent above the mean, while those with affiliations at four sites had profiles 8.2 per cent above the mean.[12] In effect, the professional responsibilities of attending physicians with admitting privileges in acute care facilities are diluted by the assumption of ancillary duties in off-site private clinics.

5 Differentiation effect

The behavioural changes noted above will, in the first instance, most directly impact on the relationship between patients and physicians. But there will also be broader, systemic impacts on medicare. Of necessity, private surgical clinics will seek to differentiate themselves from the public system by promoting a superiority of service. Indeed, it is their primary raison d'être. In the short run, this need to outperform the public system may focus on small matters such as greater comfort, privacy, and convenience. But as we have seen in the case studies above, there is an incentive to promote material changes in the standards of care as well. This differentiation effect can be expected to have two negative consequences for the public system.

First, the ability of the public system to manage demand for health care will be eroded. At present, one of the primary techniques of delivering health services for which the demand is almost infinite, with resources that are necessarily scarce, is through the development and enforcement of appropriate standards of care. If a private system, sanctioned by government, sets out to create and proclaim a higher standard of care than exists in the public system, then the latter faces one of two invidious choices. It can either raise its own standards to match the private system or it can reconcile itself to the fact that henceforward there are indeed two separate standards of treatment. The first of these choices entails unaffordable costs, and directly negates the stated rationale of permitting private operations, namely, to relieve funding pressures on the public system. The second clearly abrogates the terms of the Canada Health Act, which specify that all medically necessary services will be delivered on uniform terms and conditions.

Second, despite the assurances that queue jumping would not occur, it is evident that the introduction of a class of "enhanced" services, in which accelerated provision of treatment counts as enhancement, will precisely result in queue jumping. Indeed, this is virtually a classic case of unintended consequences waiting to happen. Consider how the dominoes have been lined up: legislation is drafted to allow private care, but only for "uninsured" services. At the same time, queue jumping for insured services is prohibited. But the opportunity to get treatment more quickly than the public system allows is one of the most significant benefits, if not in fact the only one, that private clinics offer. There is consequently an enormous incentive to redefine insured services as "uninsured," so that the prohibition on queue jumping is avoided. Bill 11 makes this possible by the introduction of a new class of "enhanced" services. Result: the prohibition on queue jumping, intended to keep insured services out of the commercial arena, has the exact opposite effect. Indeed, we might observe that the commercial future of surgical facilities is now tied directly to their success in making progressive inroads on the public system through the methodology offered by Bill 11.

6 Market fragmentation and "creaming"
Medicare is currently paid for out of general tax revenues, rather than on a fee-for-service basis. The immediate basis for this methodology is to remove ability to pay from consideration in deciding who should receive necessary services. But there are deeper

considerations. First, ill health is largely a random and unpredictable event. It makes sense to insure against this by spreading the risk over the broadest possible pool of at-risk individuals. This opportunity, however, is diminished if the pool is subdivided among individuals with varying degrees of risk. If those who conceive themselves less likely to become ill are allowed to leave the broader pool and make their own arrangements, the relative cost of insuring the remaining group increases. In this regard, we should note the behaviour of some health insurance agencies in the United States, which refuse to insure certain at-risk professions. "Creaming" of the risk pool, which is neither open to, nor of interest to, a public health care system, develops a viability when private delivery organizations are permitted to operate on a selective basis. A similar situation develops when private automobile insurance companies are permitted to operate in jurisdictions served by public insurance systems. Frequently, the private operator signs up clients on the basis of long accident-free records and good health status, thereby creaming the market for low-cost clients. The public system is left to bear the cost of insuring the remainder of the population. While it may be reasonable to allow drivers with good records to benefit financially, the policy objective of allowing individuals with good genetic profiles to benefit in the same way is less clear.

Second, general taxation will remain a sustainable means of paying for a costly service like medicare only so long as all taxpayers conceive themselves likely to be beneficiaries at some point in their lives. If individuals within the tax pool are permitted to make their own private arrangements, even if these are initially only for some limited category of services, the viability of a tax-based system is diminished to that same degree. Analogously, the public education system in California found that, once a critical mass of parents had been allowed to remove their children from the state-run system and enroll them in private schools, public support for K-12 education through the state tax system was greatly weakened.

Consequently, it is reasonable to expect that if people are allowed to begin purchasing adjunct care, it is only a matter of time before they will protest at paying for the costs of others. Again, contrary to the assumption that permitting private care to develop will relieve funding pressures on the public system, we may anticipate that public funding will in fact be imperilled by permitting private payment arrangements.

7 Patient impacts

The impacts discussed above are mainly associated either with changes in physician practice, or with broader attitudinal changes at the general population level. However, there are also likely to be impacts on patient outlook and behaviour. Perhaps the most profound impact is likely to come from the realization that the physician providing treatment now has interests that diverge from that of the patient. In other kinds of interaction, this would not necessarily be of concern. Someone shopping for a new car or a lawn mower or a pound of steak knows that his interests and those of the potential vendors do not coincide. He also knows, or has available to him, the means of protecting his own interests. He can shop around, compare prices, lower his expectations, or put off the purchase entirely if circumstances are unfavourable.

None of these means of protection is reasonably available to someone who needs medical treatment. There is a huge imbalance between the level of knowledge of the patient and that of the care provider. This is further reflected in a status and power configuration that greatly enhances the position of the latter in regard to the former. One of the fundamental objectives of medical due process in the public health system is to prevent this imbalance working to the detriment of patients.

Anxiety, fear, and guilt are also significant factors in the mindset of patients and their families faced with making a financial decision about medical treatment. These factors are so significant that it is often remarked that health care, if treated as a commodity, does not "trade." That is, it is impossible to establish a viable market system in which purchaser and seller interact in a balanced or sustainable manner.

Notwithstanding these concerns, Bill 11 permits patients who enter a surgical facility with the expectation of receiving an insured service to be billed for other enhanced or non-medical goods and services, so long as the nature of these charges is explained in advance by the physician and agreed to in writing by the patient. This provision would appear to afford considerable potential for miscommunication at best, and exploitation at worst. The following anecdote may offer some insight into the probable consequences of this provision.

Some years ago the Government of Saskatchewan, looking for a way to bring home to people the real costs of health care, sent to each resident of the province a detailed account of the costs incurred over the last year in providing health services to that resident. The material was liberally punctuated with statements to the effect that this was not in any sense a bill, but simply an information piece for the benefit of the reader. Despite this, the Department of Health was sent cheques by mail, often from senior citizens, in the belief that they owed the amount indicated in the material they had received. Other provinces have reported similar experiences.

But there is a deeper sense in which we must expect people's sense of identity and social being to be altered by the introduction of commercial values into health administration. Presently, the equality of medical treatment that medicare aims at resonates deeply with the instinctive urge of Canadians for equality and fair treatment in all aspects of civic life. It is unlikely that the visible emergence, over time, of a deep-seated inequality in the provision of health services, even if this is initially constrained to services at the margin, will leave untouched those deeper values that support Canadian society.

We have seen, then, that it is reasonable to expect the development of a private system of health care delivery to lead to alterations in the behaviour of both caregivers and patients. We have also seen that several discrete mechanisms exist through which these attitudinal and behavioural changes can lead to alterations in the system of medical due process that sustains medicare. Altered practice patterns and attitudes among physicians are perhaps the most powerful factors at work. But a network of other, more subtle, behaviour changes can be identified that will also affect the viability of the public system.

Perhaps more surprisingly, we have also seen that several of the attitudinal and behavioural shifts that may be expected to occur with the introduction of a private system of care lead to outcomes directly contrary to the objectives of the privatization approach. We have seen that altered physician practice patterns may not result in any relieving of pressure on the public system, and may actually increase it. We have also seen that the economic realities of competition and product differentiation must certainly lead to pressure on the public system either to abandon self-discipline or to accept an inferior status. We have seen that whereas queue jumping is theoretically forbidden by Bill 11, it is virtually assured by the need of private facilities to occupy effectively the narrow share of the health market ceded to them. And, finally, we have seen that it is highly unlikely that patients will be able to play the role of informed purchaser that Bill 11 anticipates. It is far more probable that patients will become the undiscriminating targets of a heightened level of sales tactics in the health product field, with disturbing consequences for demand management in the public system.

For these reasons, we believe that the privatization solution to health reform will be no more successful than the orthodox approach. Whereas the orthodox initiative failed because it imposed an unworkably complex new model, the privatization solution fails because its proponents have not taken account of the impact on medical due process in the existing public system. These impacts derive from classic Foucauldian sources: the effect of institutional changes on the behaviour of individuals.

CHAPTER TWELVE

A New Approach to Managing Health Services in Canada

We have argued that health care presents unique challenges to planners and managers. This is in part because of the huge number of variables involved. If the delivery of health care is conceived as the functioning of one large, organic system, the sheer size and complexity of the resulting model renders it unpredictable at the level of detail required by managers, in the same way that meteorologists cannot predict the path of a tornado or where a hurricane will come ashore. It is also because, unlike inanimate systems such as the weather, the variables in health care systems, namely, people, act in ways that are not law-governed. As a result, attempts to manage health care as an integrated system have failed. No model in practice could handle that many interactions, and no model in principle could handle that many human interactions. We have also argued that the privatization approach favoured by the governments of Alberta and Ontario will destabilize medicare because it threatens to disrupt the internal dynamics of the public system. Privatization threatens to alter the established patterns of medical due process by which the public system preserves such fundamental values as accessibility, equality, and uniformity of treatment.

Yet health care delivery in Canada today is a $55 billion undertaking, employing hundreds of thousands of staff and operating sophisticated facilities with state-of-the-art equipment. If the reform efforts to date have not worked, the solution to the medicare crisis cannot conceivably be to renounce managing altogether and hope for the best. What is required is a new set of management principles specifically adapted to the circumstances of health care delivery. In this chapter, we offer some views as to how such a set of principles can be constructed.

Now, it is worth pausing for a moment to consider what we mean when we talk about "managing" the health care system. The term "management" has several different applications. There is a personal application of the term, in which someone may talk about managing an issue or problem that has arisen in his or her life, by which is meant taking the personal steps needed to deal with it. There is a supervisory use of the term, in which someone with administrative authority directs the work of subordinates. And there is an executive application of the term, in which a person or body with oversight authority establishes policies and parameters within which operational decisions must be taken by subordinate authorities. This latter usage resembles Foucault's use of the term "government."

The form of management we are interested in is the third of these uses, namely, executive management. It is primarily at this level that provincial governments function in respect to managing the health system. What then does executive management actually entail? Principally, it involves two discrete tasks that have to do, respectively, with defining means and ends. The challenge facing executive managers lies less in carrying out a task themselves, than in shaping the task and creating a viable operating environment in which others can carry it out. This requires first that goals be articulated in terms that correspond to the operational realities of the situation. The goals selected must be clear and coherent in themselves, and they should delineate a meaningful, achievable task for the organizational structure that must carry them out. Second, it is necessary that whatever working methodologies and administrative policies are adopted be matched in a realistic fashion with the capabilities of the operating agency that must carry them out.

In this sense, the challenge facing executive managers is primarily the conceptual task of articulating achievable objectives, and then pairing them up with an operating model capable of achieving them. And it is in designing a conceptually viable model of health care delivery that health planners and reformers have signally failed. First, in defining the task, they chose to conceive of the health care system as an organic whole, possessing functional cohesion and hence susceptible of direction at that level. This arose in part from the goals that were set, several of which – like the integration of levels of care – are most easily expressed in broad, system-wide terms. It also arose from a belief that the previous system had failed precisely because it was fragmented and lacked unity. The objectives of health reform were therefore conceptualized in terms that seemed to require an amalgamated, organizationally unified model of delivery.

Second, in designing operating methodologies to achieve these objectives, health planners chose to impose a command and control model based on orthodox business theory. This involved the introduction of a vertically structured management hierarchy penetrating all of the operating sectors of health care, and entailing large-scale management of people and their lives. It is important to understand the operational implications of this decision. As we noted earlier, the most complex decision-making structure prior to health reform was the acute care hospital. In such a body, most operational decisions were taken by staff working within sight of one another. Where policy decisions were required, they could be rendered immediately through one layer (or at most two layers) of management. While the difficulties of unpredictable human behaviour were still present, they were minimized by a number of factors. First, the staff knew one another personally, and could modify their own actions on the basis of how a colleague was seen to respond. Second, most issues arose within the four walls of the institution, and had been dealt with in one form or another before: there was a large area of common ground. Third, the institution was tightly focused – it had relatively few goals and everyone knew what these were and how their work related to them. Fourth, staff gained security from the presence of stable and knowable boundaries around them. This allowed an element of routine to emerge, through which employees were able to conserve their emotional energies. Unpredictability remained, but it was reduced to manageable proportions.

The decision to amalgamate all health care delivery agencies in one large vertically layered authority disabled many of these coping devices, and introduced additional difficulties of its own. Workplace decisions were now processed through a multitude of layers, some of which, by necessity, had to be off-site. Staff could not know these new levels of managers, and had no chance to gain familiarity with their preferences or idiosyncrasies. Tight and narrow focus was replaced with vague, far-reaching goals that extended well beyond the work site. The ability to rely on routine was disrupted, as external factors intruded that could not easily be tracked or foreseen. From the perspective of front-line workers, the sense of knowability evaporated, to be replaced with tension and frustration. From the perspective of executive management, unbridgeable gaps were opened up between the goals they set out to achieve, the measures they adopted to achieve them, and the actual outcomes that resulted.

How then should we proceed to recast the management challenge of medicare in terms susceptible of a different kind of solution? We take as our starting-point the principal system improvements that it is apparent from the current medicare crisis are essential. For simplicity, we believe these can be narrowed down to the following "big three." These are the "deliverables" that any successful approach to health care planning and management must secure.

1 *It is essential that the entitlements enshrined in medicare be restated in unambiguous terms, so that the public, health care workers, and decision makers know clearly what their rights and responsibilities are.*
2 *The operational model of health service delivery must be simplified in order to remove the endemic confusion, complexity, and layering of the current system. Meaningful efficiencies must be found in the new delivery model, and once found, maintained over time.*
3 *A means must be found to bring primary care into a more effective working relationship with the rest of the health network.*

So how can these urgent improvements be pursued without repeating the systematic failures of the past? It is apparent that we can never fully remove every aspect of unpredictability. An irreducible amount of unforeseen, random behaviour will remain no matter what precautions we adopt. Rather, we believe the solution is to search for a design model that minimizes these factors. We begin this process by drawing attention to the specific operating features of the current reform approach that we believe must be eliminated.

First, the explicit drive toward organizational complexity and convolution inherent in the orthodox approach must be reversed. Organizations become more complex as layers of decision making are added, as multiple goals are embraced, as the number of stakeholders with a say in any given decision increases, and as operating units with quite different conditions for success are mixed together or merged. Complexity is also increased as managers turn to external consultants and advisers for input into decision making. Health reform, as a matter of deliberate policy, set out to foster and enjoin all of these occurrences. Indeed, it might reasonably be said that the primary instrument of health reform – regionalization – was expressly designed to increase the complexity of the health care system, on the premise that the original delivery structure was too primitive and narrowly focused to pursue the higher-order goals of health planners. The unspoken, and unsupported, assumption was made that if greater horizontal integration of services was required, the way to get there was by imposing a complex, vertical delivery model. We believe this unspoken assumption was incorrect and should now be discarded.

The second characteristic of health planning that has contributed to failure has been the tendency to impose top-down solutions that rely on the enforcement of conformity and compliance, rather than models that favour soliciting co-operation by increments. This tendency can be seen most readily in the way regionalization was imposed (usually by *force majeure* on reluctant independent operators) in the way clinical practice guidelines are developed at arm's-length from the medical profession, or in way primary care reform is proceeding. But it can also be observed in the way the Canadian public has been excluded from any meaningful involvement in decision making around the key choices confronting medicare. In part, the reason for adopting this top-down model has been the prevailing sense of urgency among decision makers. In part, it results from frustration at what many politicians and health planners see as obduracy on the part of physician groups and health unions. In part, it may also reflect a pervasive refusal by the Canadian public to face realities. In an August 2000 Angus Reid poll, conducted for the Canadian Medical Association, 83 per cent of respondents said they would favour relieving pressure on the health system by reallocating funds from other government programs or raising taxes. No government in the country believes the public would actually support such a solution were it to be implemented

A third characteristic of health care reform that we believe has contributed to failure has been the refusal of provincial decision makers to create a reasonable degree of clarity around the core entitlements of medicare. Not a single provincial Treasury Board, when setting the health care budget, has before it either a schedule of services that meet the test of "medical necessity," and are therefore protected by medicare, or a list of service levels that satisfy the requirement of "reasonableness" and must therefore be funded. Instead, the basic deliverables of medicare are arm-wrestled behind closed doors, without either a road map to guide the discussion or a meaningful process of public involvement to sustain it. The result has been a series of incremental budget cuts, peripheral lopping, and localized exigency measures that have added greatly to the public sense of bewilderment and dismay. We are not referring to the occasional breakdowns in communication or accidental misdirections that can happen in any field. The issue is rather systemic ambiguity, in which the delivery model is subjected over time to so many piecemeal, inconsistent, and even contradictory changes that it becomes impossible to form a clear picture from those messages or signals that do get through to the front lines.

As a result, a sense of inaccessibility has grown up around the way health care decisions are being made, in which the public feels marginalized and powerless to influence events. The only certainty in such a situation is that those at the front line, whether caregivers or patients, will see the situation differently than the planners and managers who are responsible for determining broad policy direction. This is not just an indictment of the way a vital area of public policy has been conducted. It is a sure and certain recipe for failure.

The final characteristic of health reform that has led to failure has been the repeated tendency of health planners to mistake heuristic models for operational plans. Theoretical constructs useful only for illustrative purposes have been converted into the blueprints for actual organizational entities. As a result, a delivery model emerged that is completely dysfunctional in operational terms. From the perspective of management, this model provided no predictive capability at the work-site level, where management decisions must actually take effect. From the perspective of staff, the model created a nonviable work environment in which vital coping mechanisms are disabled by scale and complexity.

Let us now consider how a different management approach might be constructed that could achieve the "big three" deliverables while, so far as possible, eliminating or reducing the undesirable systems features we have identified. We look first at the challenge of reclarifying the basic entitlements of medicare. It is our view that this responsibility rests principally with the federal government. We discussed earlier the political and constitutional reasons that prevented Ottawa from spelling out in the medicare legislation precisely what rights and duties were entailed. This has provided a fertile source of much of the confusion and obfuscation that surrounds medicare today. We believe that the Parliament of Canada now has the responsibility to correct this state of affairs, notwithstanding which level of government may have operational authority.

The challenge for Ottawa, given the constitutional division of powers, is to find a way to articulate in greater detail the rights and duties of both users and providers of health services in Canada. It will be remembered that in the Canada Health Act, the route chosen was to set out a framework of broad principles, such as universality and accessibility, and then to introduce a series of operational stipulations, including the requirements that health services be publicly administered and delivered in a uniform manner. Ottawa's purpose in specifying these particular operational requirements was to ensure that the provinces, while acting independently of one another, would in fact create a viable national health service. Absent the constitutional authority to impose these operational factors, the federal government instead made transfer payments conditional on their adoption. By this mechanism, compliance was secured.

We believe that the recent trend of judicial intervention and decision making in the field of health care rights suggests a means whereby the federal government can now act to clarify health care rights. Specifically, it now appears possible for the federal government to amend the Canada Health Act by incorporating a medicare charter that spells out in greater detail the principal rights and duties of both users and providers of health services in Canada. We believe this course of action is open to Ottawa because, as we have seen, the effect of a series of recent court rulings has been to bring health care entitlements within the protection of the Charter of Rights and Freedoms. So long as the Parliament of Canada is acting to give further definition and procedural protection to rights guaranteed under the Canadian Charter, it seems likely that such legislation would withstand a constitutional challenge. However, even if the constitutional position is not yet fully clear, it would be open to the federal government to employ the device of conditional funding to gain compliance. Failing even this contingency, we believe it remains a fundamental responsibility of Parliament to clarify its own views with respect to such a key public policy matter as the health care rights of Canadians.

In this respect, it should be noted that the UK has done detailed work on a Patients Charter for the NHS in the last ten years. Among the rights included in the present UK version are the following:

- Respect for privacy, dignity, and religious and cultural beliefs
- Freedom in choosing, and changing, a GP
- Full access to personal health records
- Right to a full and prompt written reply regarding any complaint
- Right to treatment at out-patient clinics and emergency facilities within stated time limits

- Appointment of a named nurse responsible for the patient's nursing care while in hospital
- Assurance that if a scheduled operation is cancelled twice, the patient will be admitted within one month of the second cancellation

In practical terms, these rights are a combination of basic values, such as respect for privacy and freedom of choice, and specific treatment standards, such as policies for rescheduling operations and acceptable waiting times at emergency facilities. In the Canadian federal system of government, one might expect the former to reside in a national charter, while the latter would be more appropriate at the provincial level. Interestingly, though the language of "patient charters" has not been used, Ottawa is currently pressing the provinces to adopt published standards of performance in exchange for increased federal funding.

There is no point, however, in the federal government merely pressing the provinces to formalize their own current treatment standards. This will simply set in concrete the fragmented, piecemeal state of affairs that currently besets medicare. Yet, as we write, this is precisely what Ottawa is proposing to do. The Prime Minister has conceded to the premiers of Ontario and Quebec that whatever national standards are adopted can be based on those standards already in place in each province. Not only is this an abdication of federal responsibilities to maintain a genuine national framework for health care entitlements, but the process embodies everything that is wrong with decision making in this field. There has been no public consultation, discussions are conducted in an atmosphere of political log-rolling, and an air of urgency pervades.

What is urgently required is for Ottawa instead to proclaim its own set of national standards for medicare in Canada, and to do so in unambiguous, principled terms. Since neither of us is a legislative drafter, we present below in purely schematic terms an outline of how Ottawa might draft such a Canadian medicare charter.

SECTION 1: VALUES AND PRINCIPLES

Health services in Canada shall continue to be provided in a manner consistent with the following principles:

- Universality: All of the residents in each province are entitled to receive medicare services on uniform terms and conditions.

- Comprehensiveness: Medicare will provide all medically necessary services carried out by hospitals, medical practitioners, or dentists, and similar or additional services rendered by other health care practitioners.
- Accessibility: Medicare services must be provided on uniform terms and conditions, and on a basis that does not impede or preclude, either directly or indirectly, whether by charges or otherwise, access to these services.
- Portability: Medicare will provide the same services in all regions and provinces of Canada.
- Public administration: Medicare will continue to be publicly administered.

SECTION 2: OPERATING PRACTICES

- A national registry of essential medical services will be established by the federal government, in consultation with the provinces. A board of directors, representative of each region and province of Canada, will oversee the registry, and a professional staff will be appointed to carry out its mandate.
- All medical services, or categories of service, deemed by the national registry to be essential shall be provided to all Canadians, in all provinces and territories, as publicly operated medicare services, and no charge shall be levied for their provision in any facility.
- Effective access to a general practitioner should be available to all Canadians in a non-emergency, community facility on a twenty-four-hour basis.
- Every citizen should have the right to choose and to change their general practitioner.
- All medicare services will be administered on a not-for-profit basis by a public authority appointed or designated by the government of the province.
- Privately operated facilities may provide non-essential treatments: they may also provide essential treatments on an out-patient basis, providing that the terms and conditions of treatment do not differ from those of the public system.
- Every health care provider, including physicians, nurses, and medical specialists, has the right to choose whether to work in a public or a private facility, but may not work simultaneously in both.
- Every health care provider has the right to work in a safe environment.

We believe that a clarification of rights, framed in the kind of language suggested above, meets the evolving test of constitutional authority within which the federal government must operate. Specifically, the enhanced definitions of due process requirements contained in this statement are consistent with recent indications of judicial thinking about health care rights. We believe that the federal government can make a strong showing that Canada's experience operating a public health care system now justifies a stronger articulation of rights and due process than was contained in the original statutes.

We turn now to the second management challenge that a new approach to health reform must meet, namely, reintroducing a level of functional simplicity and clarity in the delivery apparatus of medicare and achieving meaningful efficiency savings. We believe it is essential at this point to confront an unpleasant reality. This is that regionalization, the centrepiece of orthodox health reform, has failed. Rather than capturing economies of scale as intended, regionalization has led instead to the increased ability of health delivery agencies to resist change. In a process akin to fortification, the walls simply grew higher. We would also observe that the merger of operating units with such widely differing conditions for success and staff esprit as intensive care units, birthing suites, home care services, senior citizen housing units, laundry operations, banking and insurance functions, groundskeeping, and building maintenance makes the search for economy and efficiency more rather than less difficult. For those techniques that are most conducive of economy in one area may be least applicable in another. Concentration of effort and unity of purpose, perhaps the two most important requirements of managing change, are almost disabled when organizational coherence dissolves in a welter of unrelated priorities and tribalistic turf protecting. Moreover, the improved health outcomes that regionalization promised to deliver have been swamped by the turmoil, anger, and alienation that reform has let loose. The complexity of the model, in practical operating terms, is so formidable that mere survival, rather than the introduction of change, has become the order of the day for managers and health care workers.

We also believe, for the reasons given in chapter 11, that the privatization option favoured by the Government of Alberta poses an unacceptable degree of risk to our public health delivery system. It appears highly unlikely that this option can be implemented without provoking a series of unintended and unfortunate consequences, both for medicare and for the private system itself.

Consequently the correct solution, regrettably given the expenditures of effort to date, is to return to a simpler management model of health service delivery in which organizational coherence can be re-established. This is not the omnibus, multi-function, multi-site, multi-service regional health authority that most provinces have created. Rather, it implies a scaled-down delivery structure in which unity of purpose and congruity of professional patterns of practice form the boundaries. We believe this can be achieved as follows.

First, regional health authorities should be divided into two distinct functional components: a support division that provides administrative or "hotel" services, and a delivery division that provides care. The first division would include administration, personnel, finance and insurance, laundry, food preparation, building maintenance, housekeeping, and possibly some routine, high-volume functions such as basic lab tests that are machine-read and some components of X-ray processing. A common feature of all these functions is that they offer economies of scale if these are aggressively pursued. The National Forum on Health Care recently reported that savings of one-third of all health expenditures could be achieved without impairing quality or accessibility of care. It is our own view that there remains a significant potential for economies to be found well away from the bed side, in the 25 to 30 per cent of acute and long-term care budgets that are devoted to the so-called "hotel services." Some means must be devised to put these resources to better use. Experience with regional authorities, however, has shown that the economies available have not, in fact, been pursued aggressively. No doubt this is due in part to the difficulty of introducing functions such as automation, off-site delivery, and mass production into an organization structured around the delivery of health care. Health authorities have also found that it is difficult to negotiate with powerful health unions on their home turf.

We believe the solution lies in turning these functions over to private operators, through a competitive bidding process. Health authorities would retain the functions related to contract management, which would include designing specifications to meet dietary necessities, special laundry requirements (for instance, long-term care residents need softer sheets), and so on. But the actual production work would be privatized, and often completed off-site. By using private operators to do this work, the element of competition is introduced into at least one aspect of health care delivery.

The second division includes those services involved in the direct delivery of care to patients. These include all of the remaining functions of acute and long-term care, home care, and primary care. We believe what is required is an organizational structure in which most direct decision making regarding the care of individual patients is returned to the facility level, that is to say, to the hospital, long-term care facility, or community clinic level. This is the traditional organizational unit within which most health care providers are used to working and having decisions made. The goal should be that most or all clinical treatment decisions should be made no greater than two organizational layers from the bedside. Decisions made outside this level would be restricted to the following categories:

- Annual budgets
- Patient transfers
- Utilization policies

These would be developed by interdisciplinary committees representing the various levels of care, and confirmed by the regional board. By this means, improved integration of care and other systemic goals could still be pursued, but based on teamwork and collaboration rather than a command and control model. Central coordination of these activities would be supplied by a secretariat function, reporting through a general manager to the regional board. Corporate titles such as "chief executive officer" and "vice-president" would be replaced with the traditional health sector titles of "administrator" and "nurse manager." By this means, the multi-layered bureaucracies characteristic of most regional health authorities would be replaced by small coordinating secretariats. Clinical decision making would be restored to the facility level, and routine support functions would be privatized.

It is also important to consider the role of provincial governments in restoring a functional decision-making model in health care delivery. It is a fundamental necessity of health service delivery that a locus of decision making exist with the authority to render a clear decision around genuinely global issues. First and foremost, this includes the ability and willingness to set some practical limit on the availability of resources. Yet this is no simple matter. It has been found over the last twenty years that public health care systems exhibit a variant of Parkinson's law: left unchecked, they expand to consume all available resources. This is due in part to the open-endedness of the goals aimed at in the health field: you can never have "too much" good health. It results also from the chemistry of interaction between patients and physicians. The patient is not an informed or "rational" decision maker in the sense used by economists, while the physician tends to lack the professional or financial motivation to act as a moderating force. Commercial pressures from pharmaceutical suppliers, equipment manufacturers, and so on also add to the demands for increased health spending.

In the commercial sector, the device used to balance supply with demand is the price mechanism. With limited exceptions, such a mechanism is not presently available to regulate the supply of health services. Consequently, it is a basic requirement of managing the health sector that an effective decision-making centre be created with both the authority and the will to limit resources. Moreover, this authority must be exercised in a manner consistent with the basic rights of Canadians to equality and accessibility in health service delivery, or we must expect the courts to invalidate whatever decisions are taken.

How then should a decision-making centre with the authority and will power to limit resources conduct itself? The first observation we can make is that decisions, when they are given, must emerge through some process comprehensible to and supportable by both health care professionals and the public. This is certainly not how health care funding decisions have been made in Canada over the last twenty years. The process used has been ad hoc, secretive, and heavily dependent on the use of diversionary tactics such as Fed-bashing by the provinces and grandstanding by Ottawa.

Moreover, the challenge is more than to say "no" in a way that does not appear simply arbitrary or ad hoc. As noted earlier, the estimate by a provincial/territorial working group that baseline health spending will grow by almost 250 per cent over the next twenty-five years makes no allowance for the emergence of new diseases or new technologies. Now, experience shows that over time, as a new technology gains acceptance and its application becomes widespread, marginal prices usually stabilize and may even fall. This happens as the production base expands, economies of scale arise, and clinicians gain familiarity with the new device or procedure. What we must be concerned with is not the prospect of emergent new technology per se: the real challenge to sustainability lies in the prospect of a significant expansion of the rate at which new technologies become available. Many believe that the onset of genetic re-engineering, offering not just new treatments but a genuinely different approach to clinical interventions, represents just such a challenge. Some observers have gone so far as to predict that the genetic "revolution" will equal the discovery of antibiotics and the introduction of anaesthetics in its power to reshape medical science.

It appears possible then that a decision-making capability may be required that can not only limit resources, but that has the discipline to refuse funding for at least some new treatments that may be efficacious. This represents the emergence of an ethical and management dilemma essentially new to health policy. For most of the history of health care delivery, the challenge was to find new cures and make them available. More recently, when unaffordable budget demands by the health sector led to cuts in programs and service levels, it was still possible for health managers to point to significant overutilization of many services as the justification for budget cutting. But what is in prospect now is a surge of new technologies, and new cost pressures, that may overwhelm any credible effort to reassign existing resources. We would note that the rapid expansion of the Internet is likely to add to the pressure, as knowledge of potential new treatments is diffused throughout the broader population. In effect, the possibility is raised that a form of medical triage may have to be elevated to state policy. This surely raises the stakes enormously, both for decision makers and for the public.

How then should a decision centre be structured to make the kinds of difficult decisions that may be required of it? We believe it is essential that key decisions that touch on fundamental entitlements be taken through some form of adjudicative process that has administrative, if not policy, independence from government. It is impractical to remove decisions about one-third or more of government budgets from the financial oversight of provincial treasury boards and cabinets, but it is possible to delegate matters having to do with standards of treatment and medical due practice. Most provincial government operate medical services commissions that might perform these responsibilities. A viable structure can be created by appointing a tripartite board, comprising medical experts, members of the public, and senior government managers to oversee the work of the commission. So long as the mandate of such a commission is properly balanced, it is possible for government to delegate specific clinical or treatment matters without losing overall budget control.

Let us consider how this process might function, by examining how a real-life decision was made, and then applying this new methodology. In 1997, the Government of British Columbia was asked to fund, as a medicare-insured service, the provision of deaf interpretation services for patients whose physical disability prevented them from communicating with their physicians.[1] We take our interpretation of the case from the Court's written judgment. The government declined to fund interpretation services, arguing that deafness was a condition of the claimants that had nothing to do with the health scheme and that, in refusing interpreters, the health plan treated the deaf and non-deaf equally. At this point, the options facing the claimants were limited. They could either accept the situation or launch a court challenge. They took the latter route, and the British Columbia Supreme Court found in their favour. In a judgment that was later upheld by the Supreme Court of Canada, the Court instructed the government to fund sign language interpreters as a medical service.

We believe that a decision-making process of this kind does everyone involved a disservice. While government officials often have good reasons for their judgments, it can be difficult to establish these in the somewhat one-sided situations that must emerge when largely uninformed citizens plead their case with expert government consultants. It can also be difficult for the public to accept an adverse judgment, when the decision rests solely with harried or busy officials who must balance many other interests. We would argue that situations of this kind could better be adjudicated if they were taken before a medical services commission, sitting in public session. This would allow for the presentation of issues in a more objective or balanced environment, because the tripartite nature of the commission incorporates professional and lay opinion, as well as government views. By introducing an element of due process, this approach also ensures procedural fairness. We suspect that in most cases the same outcome would occur as happens when officials simply make a decision. But it would be a decision more comprehensible to the public, and hence more acceptable. It is also more likely that a decision rendered in this environment would withstand a court challenge, were this subsequently to occur.

One can imagine that governments might hesitate to take such a step, fearing a torrent of special pleading. But, in fact, much of this advocacy occurs at present; it simply occurs out of the public domain. Moreover, it should not be necessary for a medical services commission, structured as suggested, to grant hearings in all circumstances. A summary process would remain available for cases without evident merit, or for cases already disposed of by precedent. Moreover, inconvenient though such a prospect might seem to governments, it offers a more manageable approach than waiting for the courts to intervene. Most importantly, we would argue that as the concept of health care as a right takes shape, some form of specially developed due process is the only sustainable way to adjudicate the inevitable disputes that will arise.

We turn now to the third management challenge: bringing primary care into a more effective working alignment with the rest of the health care sector. We believe that the real challenge here lies in gaining professional support for whatever measures are implemented. In fields such as remuneration reform or the development of clinical practice guidelines, there is enough research already in place to form the basis of whatever specific policies are adopted. The problem to date is that much of the research, and almost all of the policy shaping, occurs outside the formal representative bodies of the profession. We present our suggestions below.

First, the process of developing guidelines or standards must be reunited with the internal methodologies of the medical profession through which new standards of care are constantly assessed and promulgated. This would help to avoid the virtual debacle that has befallen the guidelines initiative in the us, in which a growing number of physicians see guidelines as mere cookie-cutter devices dreamt up by HMOs to keep costs down. But if the solution is to involve the medical profession in the development of guidelines, how is this to be done? In Canada at the present time responsibility for the development of standards of care rests with the profession. These standards evolve slowly over time, often in response to new technologies, such as the laparoscope, or new drug therapies. Responsibility for developing these standards is distributed in a somewhat ill-defined manner, with provincial colleges of physicians and surgeons, medical associations, and university medical schools all playing a role. But final authority for pronouncing on standards, both in the case of licensure and in disciplinary matters, rests with provincial colleges.

It is our view that the locus of responsibility for developing appropriateness standards should rest at the level of provincial College of Physicians and Surgeons, given that the colleges function as the primary professional standards and adjudicative body for the profession.

To ensure that a reasonable priority and urgency is placed on the adoption of new appropriateness standards, it would be reasonable to create multidisciplinary panels within each provincial College, charged with this work. In fact, many Colleges already make use of such arrangements in the conduct of their other duties. Once appropriateness standards are agreed to by this process, the practice of continuing medical education, which physicians are required to take part in, can be used to diffuse knowledge of such standards. Computer software programs are increasingly becoming available that enable physicians to review practice guidelines in the context of deciding treatment for a given patient. It would be wise for provincial governments and medical associations to consider funding the development and distribution of some of these packages. It may be feared that this is a responsibility that many provincial Colleges will be reluctant to assume. And given current physician attitudes to guidelines, this is a likely first reaction. Yet it must be remembered that the principal concern about guidelines is not their necessity, but their parentage. If a bona fide offer were made to transfer responsibility for the development of guidelines to the profession's own standards-setting body, we believe it would be difficult if not impossible for the medical profession to decline such an offer.

It is also important that a means be found to shield clinical decision making from the undue influences of the threat of litigation. Most provinces contribute to the Canadian Medical Practices Association (CMPA) fund, which insures physicians against the cost of lawsuits for malpractice. Although it is common for provinces to dislike and seek to avoid funding CMPA, we believe that government involvement in this mechanism sends an important signal of support to the profession.

It is also clear that the family practice model must be modernized, both as regards the system of remuneration, and with respect to the isolation of primary care providers from the rest of the health care network. This issue has proved so highly contentious over the years in Canada (and elsewhere), that little or no progress has been made. A number of provinces, frustrated with this dilemma, are now considering handing the problem to regional health authorities and letting them sort it out. We can scarcely conceive of an approach more likely to fail. It is unlikely in the best of circumstances that governments could expect to succeed in imposing by force a top-down restructuring of professional practice upon physicians. It is still less likely that turning such a difficult matter over to inexperienced regional health authorities can lead to anything but complete breakdown. To revert to our earlier analogy, it is as if our riverside spectator, grown weary with just counting bodies, decides to push in a few of his own.

We believe that this is an initiative that must be rooted in the medical profession and its representative bodies, if it is to succeed. Because issues of remuneration and the structure of practice arrangements are involved, this is more a matter that provincial medical associations, in conjunction with the Canadian Medical Association, should undertake, rather than Colleges of Physicians and Surgeons. We believe that if the provinces and Ottawa approached the profession with a request that physicians themselves take the lead in designing a new set of practice principles, it would be possible to gain support for such an initiative. The chances of success would be increased if the provinces gave certain assurances at the outset, including:

- No physician in practice today will be forced to alter his or her employment status.
- The five-year budget of $1 billion for primary care reform that was established by the federal government as part of the Canada Health and Social Transfer restitution in September 200c will be used to create a series of incentives for physicians to join the new scheme, including assistance with the information systems and office arrangements required to operate more complex practice models.
- Provinces are open to a number of practice modalities, including clinic-style operations, the traditional family practice model, and clinician teams.

It is more likely that through such a collaborative approach, a solution will be found that meets the objectives of managers and health care providers. Such an approach will not likely commend itself to planners in a hurry or to exponents of top-down solutions. We believe, however, that the turmoil, anger, and failure to deliver stated goals, which have dogged the health reform process and brought medicare to its knees, entitle a different point of view to be heard.

Yet the question lingers, how did all of this come about? How did the NDP governments of provinces like Saskatchewan, Manitoba, and British Columbia, linear descendants of Tommy Douglas and Emmett Hall, come to embrace the orthodox reform program with its solutions at once so implausible and destructive? How could a public policy prescription so clearly ill suited to the needs of medicare be pressed on an icon of social democratic philosophy by those committed to uphold it?

And how could Ralph Klein and Mike Harris, the embodiments of decent pragmatism and working-class aspirations, come to flirt with quite another, but no less mischievous, expedient? In a country that prides itself that it is not the USA, how could an approach modelled on one of the most notable failures of recent American domestic policy gain credence?

In part, the answer lies in the grim experience of the 1980s and early 1990s, when the imperatives of fiscal recovery obscured all else. In part, the answer lies with those on both sides of the political ledger who saw an opportunity to pursue the parochial interests of greed and power, and seized it. But mainly, the answer lies with the numerous well-intentioned policy advisers, ministry officials, and treasury board staffs, who found comfort in complexity and who mistook a helpful metaphor for a management campaign. Foucault would have known better.

Notes

FOREWORD

1 Institute for Research on Public Policy Task Force on Health Policy, 2000.

PREFACE

1 Referring to the industrial efficiency pioneer Frederick Winslow Taylor, 1856–1915.

CHAPTER ONE

1 We use "agent" in a broad sense that includes administrators, physicians, nurses, paramedics, nurses' aides, technicians, and other health care providers.
2 Our exposition of Foucault is based primarily on Prado 1995 and 2000.
3 Institutional methods that effect "meticulous control of the operations of the body ... might be called 'disciplines'"; Foucault 1979: 137. Discipline's end is "the obedient subject, the individual subjected to habits, rules, orders, an authority that is exercised continually around him and upon him"; Foucault 1979: 128–9.
4 Foucault 1983: 208–9.
5 Foucault 1983: 208–9.
6 The shift from genealogy to ethics is problematic. Foucault's self-determining ethics require awareness of how discipline shapes us, but genealogy makes "[g]enuine self-knowledge ... in a sense impossible, since the self that we make appear to ourselves as an object of knowledge will never be identical to the self that is constructing that object"; Hoy 1988: 16.
7 See, for instance, Sawicki 1991.

8 Rorty 1989: 63.
9 Foucault 1979: 135–228.
10 Foucault 1979: 26.
11 Foucault 1979: 187.

1 Power is "a question of government" for Foucault, in "the very broad meaning which it had in the Sixteenth Century"; Foucault 1983: 221. The archaic sense of "government" was more inclusive than the current sense that refers mainly to "political structures or the management of states." The old term "designated the way in which the conduct of individuals ... might be directed"; Foucault 1983: 221.
2 In *Madness and Civilization*, Foucault maintains that madness was *invented* by compiling behavioural idiosyncrasies into manifestations of theoretical psychological disorders.
3 Foucault 1980a: 95.
4 Foucault 1980a: 93.
5 Foucault 1983: 219–20.
6 Foucault 1983: 219–20.
7 Foucault 1980a: 97.
8 Foucault 1980a: 94. "Nonsubjective" power has no point of view, as does some one's or some group's power in the ordinary sense.
9 Foucault 1983: 219–20.
10 It bears repeating that power is not force exerted by individuals on other individuals. Exertions of force by individuals are only power's component actions, not power itself.
11 Foucault 1983: 219–20.
12 Foucault 1980b: 93.
13 Foucault 1988: 240.
14 Foucault 1979: 138.
15 For Foucault, the "natures" that discipline serves are social constructs.
16 Rorty 1989: 63.
17 Ghettos are an intermediate step.

CHAPTER THREE

1 Wilson 1999: 91.
2 Wilson 1999: 94. At levels above the molecular, "the difficulties of synthesis are ... more difficult. Entities such as organisms and species, unlike electrons and atoms, are indefinitely variable. Worse, each ... changes during development and evolution."
3 Wilson 1999: 92–3. The tract had no cougars that preyed on seed-eating rodents. The rodent population swelled, too many seeds were

eaten, the growth of vegetation was reduced, and plant-dependent life forms died out.

4 Wilson 1999: 93.
5 *Webster's New World Encyclopedia* 1992: 225.
6 Jauhar 2000b.
7 Of course, managers and practitioners are also patients at one time or another.
8 Collins and Kusch 1998.
9 Collins and Kusch 1998: 1.
10 Wilson 1999: 95.
11 Fox-Keller 1985. The work of feminist philosophers like Evelyn Fox-Keller on the formulation of theoretical questions in science is a notable example.
12 Foucault 1983: 212.
13 Ramson 1997: 37.
14 Davidson 1986: 221.
15 Foucault 1997: 177.
16 Hacking 1986: 237.
17 Foucault 1986: 26–7.
18 Hacking 1981: 29.
19 Jauhar 2000a.
20 There is much to be said about contextual constraints. too, but our focus here is subjective constraints.
21 Jauhar 2000a.

CHAPTER FOUR

1 Even in Canada, where such advertising is restricted, pharmaceutical companies can make Web sites and phone numbers available that enable them to respond to consumer-initiated requests for information.

CHAPTER FIVE

1 Provincial and Territorial Ministers of Health 2000: 16.
2 Appleby 1999: 79–89.
3 Although inflation was lower in the 1990s, there is evidence that spending on private services increased significantly in this period.
4 Provincial and Territorial Ministers of Health 2000: 16.
5 Conference Board of Canada 2000.

CHAPTER SIX

1 DeCoster et al. 1999: 187–205.
2 Frankel, Ebrahim, and Smith 2000: 40–5.

3 They disparage as a form of sentimentality the outburst of public outrage when a health authority refused treatment to a child with non-Hodgkin's lymphoma.
4 Kohn, Corrigan, and Donaldson 2000.
5 Kohn, Corrigan, and Donaldson 2000: 50.
6 Kohn, Corrigan, and Donaldson 2000: 51.
7 Kohn, Corrigan, and Donaldson 2000: 54–5.

CHAPTER SEVEN

1 Shortell et al. 1993: 447–65.
2 Sir Roy Griffiths, Report of the National Health Service Management Enquiry, London 1983.
3 Luft 1979.
4 Wright 1997.
5 We write this in the aftermath of the Walkerton fiasco, which casts a different light on these accomplishments.
6 Krushelnicki and Belvedere 1988.
7 Provincial and Territorial Ministers of Health 2000.
8 Brossart 2000.
9 Emphasis added.
10 Cabana et al. 1999.
11 Nguyen 1996.
12 Chan et al. 1998.
13 Gruber, Kim, and Mayzlin 1999.
14 Chan et al. 1998.
15 Badgett and Rablais 1997.
16 Hutchinson et al. 1996.
17 Hurley and Labelle 1995.

CHAPTER EIGHT

1 Naylor et al. 1995.
2 Sada et al. 1998.
3 Weissman et al. 1991.
4 Hadley, Steinberg, and Feder 1991.
5 Zimmerman, Mieczjowski, and Raymond 1999.
6 Arnold and Schlenker 1992.
7 Shih 1999.
8 Furth et al. 1999.
9 Hsia et al. 2000.
10 The literature also contains reports of studies that did not find the kind of variances noted above. This appears due, in part, to study

methodology and scope. While we believe the examples quoted above are generally representative of findings in the literature, our point is simply that, to the extent these different patterns of behaviour do occur, it is due to administrative rules, not clinical decision making.

11 Dunlop, Coyte, and McIsaac 1997; McIsaac, Goel, and Naylor 2000.

CHAPTER NINE

1 World Health Organization 1960: 1.
2 Canadian Charter, 1982; s. 15 (1).
3 Supreme Court of British Columbia 2000.
4 M. v. H., 1999, 2 SCR 3 at para. 78.
5 Chaoulli and Zeliotis v. Attorney General of Quebec and Attorney General of Canada. Quebec Superior Court. 2000.
6 R. v. Edwards Books and Art Ltd [1986] 2 SCR.

CHAPTER TEN

1 Sir Thomas Holmes Sellors, Open University, 1985.
2 Committee on the Costs of Medical Care, Final Report. Washington, 1932.
3 Crichton, Hsu, and Tsang 1990.

CHAPTER ELEVEN

1 Alberta Health Care Protection Act (Bill 11) 2000, s. 1.
2 Alberta Health Care Protection Act (Bill 11) 2000, s. 3.
3 Okunade and Miles 1999.
4 Lee and Gillis 1993.
5 Zhang 1997.
6 Haber and Mitchell 1999–2000.
7 Onion et al. 1999
8 Rice et al. 1999.
9 Nesbitt et al. 1991.
10 Wynia et al. 2000.
11 Iversen 1997.
12 Miller, Welch, and Welch 1996.

CHAPTER TWELVE

1 Eldridge v. British Columbia 1997.

Bibliography

Alberta. Legislative Assembly. Alberta Health Care Protection Act (Bill 11). 4th Session, 2000.

American Medical Association. *Committee on the Costs of Medical Care*, Final Report. 1932.

American Psychiatric Association. *Diagnostic and Statistical Manual of Mental Disorders*. 2d ed. Washington, DC: American Psychiatric Association, 1968.

– *Diagnostic and Statistical Manual of Mental Disorders*. 3d ed. Washington, DC: American Psychiatric Association, 1980.

– *Diagnostic and Statistical Manual of Mental Disorders*. 3d ed., rev. Washington, DC: American Psychiatric Association, 1987.

– *Diagnostic and Statistical Manual of Mental Disorders*. 4th ed. Washington, DC: American Psychiatric Association, 1994.

Appleby, J. "Government Funding of the UK National Health Service: What Does the Historical Record Reveal?" *Journal of Health Services Research and Policy* 4, no. 2, (April 1999): 79–89.

Arnold, P.J., and T.L. Schlenker. "The Impact of Health Care Financing on Childhood Immunization Practices." *American Journal of Diseases of Children* 146, no. 6 (1992): 728–32.

Badgett, J.T., and G.P. Rabalais. "Prepaid Capitation Versus Fee-for-Service Reimbursement in a Medicaid Population." *American Journal of Managed Care* 3, no. 2 (1997): 277–82.

Brody, Jane. "Quirks, Oddities, May Be Illnesses." *The New York Times*, 4 February 1997, C1-C2.

Brossart, Bonnie. *The Impact of Preventive Home Care and Seniors Housing on Health Outcomes*. Saskatoon: Health Services Utilization and Research Commission, 2000.

Cabana, Michael D., Cynthia S. Rand, Neil R. Powe, Albert W Wu, Modena H. Wilson, Paul-André C. Abboud, and Haya R. Rubin. "Why Don't

Physicians Follow Clinical Practice Guidelines?" *Journal of the American Medical Association* 282, no. 15 (1999).

Canada. Parliament. Canadian Charter of Rights and Freedoms, 1982.

Canada. Parliament. Canada Health Act, 1984.

– Canadian Charter of Rights and Freedoms, 1982.

– Medical Care Act, 1966.

Cavell, Marcia. *The Psychoanalytic Mind: From Freud to Philosophy.* Cambridge, Mass.: Harvard University Press, 1993.

Chan, B., G.M. Anderson, and M.E. Thériault. "Fee Code Creep Among General Practitioners and Family Physicians in Ontario: Why Does the Ratio of Intermediate to Minor Assessments Keep Climbing?" *Canadian Medical Association Journal* 158, no. 6 (1998): 749–54.

– "High-Billing General Practitioners and Family Physicians in Ontario: How Do They Do It?: An Analysis of Practice Patterns of GP/FPs with Annual Billings Over $400,000." *Canadian Medical Association Journal* 158, no. 6 (1998): 741–6.

Chaoulli and Zeliotis v. Attorney General of Quebec and Attorney General of Canada. Quebec Superior Court. 2000.

Collins, Harry, and Martin Kusch. *The Shape of Action: What Humans and Machines Can Do.* Cambridge, Mass.: MIT Press, 1998.

Committee on the Costs of Medical Care. Final Report. Washington: 1932.

Conference Board of Canada. *The Future Cost of Health Care in British Columbia.* Ottawa: Conference Board of Canada, 2000.

Crichton, Anne, David Hsu, and Stella Tsang. *Canada's Health Care System: Its Organization and Funding.* Ottawa: Canadian Hospital Association Press, 1990.

Danziger, Kurt. *Constructing the Subject: Historical Origins of the Psychological Subject.* Cambridge: Cambridge University Press, 1990.

Davidson, Arnold. "Archaeology, Genealogy, Ethics." In *Foucault: A Critical Reader*, ed. David Couzens Hoy. New York: Basil Blackwell, 1986.

DeCoster, C., K.C. Carrier, S. Peterson, R. Walld, and L. MacWillian. "Waiting Times for Surgical Procedures." *Medical Care* 37, no. 6 (June 1999): 187–205.

Dreyfus, Hubert, and Paul Rabinow. *Michel Foucault: Beyond Structuralism and Hermeneutics.* With an Afterword by Michel Foucault. Brighton, Sussex: The Harvester Press, 1983.

Dunlop, S., P.C. Coyte, and W. McIsaac. "Socio-economic Status and Visits to Physicians by Adults in Ontario, Canada." *Journal of Health Services Research and Policy* 2, no. 2 (1997): 94–102.

Eldridge v. British Columbia (Attorney General). (1997), 3 SCR 624.

Foucault, Michel. *Madness and Civilization: A History of Insanity in the Age of Reason.* Trans. Richard Howard. New York: Random House, 1965.

– *The Birth of the Clinic: An Archaeology of Medical Perception.* New York: Vintage Books, 1975.

- *Discipline and Punish.* Trans. Alan Sheridan. New York: Pantheon, 1979.
- *The History of Sexuality,* vol. 1. Trans. Robert Hurley. New York: Vintage, 1980a.
- *Power/Knowledge: Selected Interviews and Other Writings,* ed. Colin Gordon. New York: Pantheon, 1980b.
- "The Subject and Power." Afterword to *Michel Foucault,* by Hubert Dreyfus and Paul Rabinow. Brighton, Sussex: The Harvester Press, 1983.
- *The Use of Pleasure.* Trans. Robert Hurley. New York: Vintage, 1986.
- *Michel Foucault: Politics, Philosophy, Culture: Interviews and Other Writings, 1977–1984,* ed. Lawrence D. Kritzman. Oxford: Blackwell's, 1988.
- "Sexuality and Solitude." In *Michel Foucault: Ethics, Subjectivity and Truth,* ed. Paul Rabinow New York: Penguin, 1997.
Fox-Keller, Evelyn. *Reflections on Gender and Science.* New Haven: Yale University Press, 1985.
Frances, Allen. Foreword to *Philosophical Perspectives on Psychiatric Diagnostic Classification,* ed. J.Z. Sadler, (O.P.) Wiggins, and M. A. Schwartz. Baltimore: Johns Hopkins University Press, 1994.
Frankel, S., S. Ebrahim, and G.D. Smith. "The Limits to Demand for Health Care." *British Medical Journal* 321 (July 2000): 40–5.
Furth, S.L., W. Hwang, A.M. Neu, B.A. Fivush, and N.R. Powe. "For-profit Versus Not-for-profit Dialysis Care for Children with End Stage Renal Disease." *Pediatrics* 104 no. 3 (1999): 519–24.
Gazzaniga, Michael. *Nature's Mind: The Biological Roots of Thinking, Emotions, Sexuality, Language, and Intelligence.* New York: Basic Books, 1992.
Gruber, J., J. Kim, and D. Mayzlin. "Physician Fees and Procedure Intensity: The Case of Cesarean Delivery." *Journal of Health Economics* 18, no. 4 (1999): 473–90.
Haber, S.G., and J.B. Mitchell. "Access to Physicians' Services for Vulnerable Medicare Beneficiaries." *Inquiry* 36, no. 4 (Winter 1999–2000): 445–60.
Hacking, Ian. "The Archaeology of Foucault." *The New York Review of Books.* Reprinted in *Foucault: A Critical Reader,* by David Couzens Hoy. New York: Basil Blackwell, 1986.
- "Self Improvement." In *Foucault: A Critical Reader,* by David Couzens Hoy. New York: Basil Blackwell, 1986.
- *Mad Travelers: Reflections on the Reality of Transient Mental Illnesses.* Charlottesville: University Press of Virginia, 1998.
- *On the Social Construction of What?* Cambridge, Mass.: Harvard University Press, 1999.
Hadley, J., E.P. Steinberg, and J. Feder. "Comparison of Uninsured and Privately Insured Hospital Patients. Condition on admission, Resource Use, and Outcome." *Journal of the American Medical Association* 265, no. 3 (1991): 374–9.
Holmes Sellors, Sir Thomas. Open University. 1985.

Hoy, David Couzens. *Foucault: A Critical Reader*. New York: Basil Blackwell, 1986.

– "Foucault: Modern or Postmodern?" *After Foucault*, ed. Jonathan Arac. New Brunswick: Rutgers University Press, 1988.

Hsia, J., E. Kemper, C. Keife, J. Zapka, S. Sofaer, M. Pettinger, D. Bowen, M. Limacher, L. Lillington, and E. Mason. "The Importance of Health Insurance as a Determinant of Cancer Screening: Evidence from the Women's Health Initiative." *Preventive Medicine* 31, no. 3 (September 2000): 261–70.

Hurley, J., and R. Labelle. "Relative Fees and the Utilization of Physicians' Services in Canada." *Health Economics* 4, no. 6 (1995): 419–38.

Hutchison, B., S. Birch, J. Hurley, J. Lomas, and F. Stratford-Devai. "Do Physician-Payment Mechanisms Affect Hospital Utilization?: A Study of Health Service Organizations in Ontario." *Canadian Medical Association Journal* 154, no. 5 (1996): 653–61.

Ignatieff, Michael. "Paradigms Lost." *Times Literary Supplement* (4 September 1987): 939–40.

Institute for research on Public Policy Task Force on Health Policy. *Recommendations to First Ministers*. Montreal: IRPP, 2000.

Iversen, T. "The Effect of a Private Sector on the Waiting Time in a National Health Service." *Journal of Health Economics* 16, no. 4 (1997): 381–96.

Jauhar, Sandeep. "More Fans for Drugs That Fight Cholesterol." Science Times section of *The New York Times*, 5 September 2000a, F1-F2.

– "Saving the Heart Can Sometimes Mean Losing the Memory." Science Times section of *The New York Times*, 19 September 2000b, F1, F4.

Kohn, Linda T., Janet M. Corrigan, and Molla S. Donaldson. *To Err Is Human: Building a Safer Health System*. Washington, DC: National Academy Press, 2000.

Krushelnicki, B.W., and T. Belvedere. "Government Reorganization in Ontario: A Comparison of Service Effectiveness and Efficiency of Regional Government." *Planning Administration* 15 (1988): 59–72.

Lee, D.W., and K. D. Gillis. "Physician Responses to Medicare Physician Payment Reform: Preliminary Results on Access to Care." *Inquiry* 30, no. 4 (Winter 1993): 417–28.

Luft, H.S., J. Bunker, and A. Enthoven. "Should Operations Be Regionalized?" *New England Journal of Medicine* 301 (1979): 1364–9.

M. v. H. 1999, 2 SCR 3 at para. 78.

McIsaac, W., V. Goel, and D. Naylor. "Socio-economic Status and the Utilization of Physicians' Services: Results from the Canadian National Population Health Survey." *Social Science and Medicine* 51, no. 1 (2000): 123–33.

Miller, M.E., W.P. Welch, and H.G. Welch. "The Impact of Practicing in Multiple Hospitals on Physician Profiles." *Medical Care* 34, no. 5 (1996): 455–62.

Naylor, C. David, Kathy Sykora, Susan B. Jaglal, Stephen Jefferson, and the Steering Committee of the Adult Cardiac Care Network of Ontario.

"Waiting for Coronary Artery Bypass Surgery: Population-based Study of 8517 Consecutive Patients in Ontario, Canada." Institute for Clinical Evaluative Sciences (ICES). *The Lancet* 346 (1995): 1605–9.

Nesbitt, T.S., J.L. Tanji, J.E. Scherger, and N.B. Kahn. "Obstetric Care, Medicaid, and Family Physicians. How Policy Changes Affect Physicians' Attitudes." *Western Journal of Medicine* 155, no. 6 (1991): 653–7.

Nguyen, N.X. "Physician Volume Response to Price Controls." *Health Policy* 35, no. 2 (1996): 189–204.

Okunade, A.A., and A.P. Miles. "Medicare Physician Payment Reform and the Utilization of Cardiovascular Procedures." *Journal of Health and Social Policy* 11, no. 1 (1999): 37–52.

Onion, D.K., D.L. Meyer, D.E. Wennberg, and D.N. Soule. "Primary Caesarean Section Rates in Uninsured, Medicaid and Insured Populations of Predominantly Rural Northern New England." *Journal of Rural Health* 15, no. 1 (Winter 1999): 108–12.

Perrow, Charles. *Normal Accidents.* New York: Basic Books, 1984.

Prado, C.G. *Starting with Foucault: An Introduction to Genealogy.* Boulder, Colo., and San Francisco: Westview Press, 1995 (1st ed.), 2000 (2d ed.).

Provincial and Territorial Ministers of Health. *Understanding Canada's Health Care Costs: Final Report.* August, 2000.

R. v. Edwards Book and Art Ltd, [1986] 2 SCR.

Ramson, John S. *Foucault's Discipline: The Politics of Subjectivity.* Durham and London: Duke University Press, 1997.

Rice, T., S.C. Stearns, D.E. Pathman, S. DesHarnais, M. Brasure, and M. Tai-Seale. "A Tale of Two Bounties: The Impact of Competing Fees on Physician Behavior." *Journal of Health Politics, Policy and Law* 24, no. 6 (1999): 1307–30.

Rorty, Richard. *Contingency, Irony, and Solidarity.* Cambridge: Cambridge University Press, 1989.

Sada, M.J., W.J. French, D.M. Carlisle, N.C. Chandra, J.M. Gore, and W.J. Rogers. "Influence of Payer Status on Use of Invasive Cardiac Procedures and Patient Outcomes After Myocardial Infarction in the United States." *Journal of the American College of Cardiology* 31, no. 7 (June 1998): 1474–80.

Sawicki, Jana. *Disciplining Foucault.* London: Routledge, 1991.

Shih, Y.C. "Effect of Insurance on Prescription Drug Use by ESRD [End Stage Renal Disease] Beneficiaries." *Health Care Financing Review* 20. no. 3 (Spring 1999): 39–54.

Shortell, S.M., R.R. Gillies, D.A. Anderson, J.B. Mitchell, and K.L. Morgan. "Creating Organized Delivery Systems: The Barriers and Facilitators." *Hospital Health Service Administration* 38 (1993): 447–65.

Showers, Carolin, Lyn Abramson, and Michael Hogan. "The Dynamic Self: How the Content and Structure of the Self-concept change with Mood." *Journal of Personality and Social Psychology* 75 (1998): 478–93.

Siever, Larry, and William Frucht. *The New View of Self: How Genes and Neu-rotransmitters Shape Your Mind, Your Personality, and Your Mental Health.* New York: MacMillan, 1997.

Supreme Court of British Columbia. Auton et al. v. the Attorney General of British Columbia and the Medical Services Commission of British Columbia. April 2000.

Webster's New World Encyclopedia. New York: Prentice-Hall, 1992, 225.

Weissman, J.S., R. Stern, S.L. Fielding, and A.M. Epstein. "Delayed Access to Care: Risk Factors, Reasons and Consequences." *Annals of Internal Medicine* 114, no. 4 (February 1991): 325–31.

Wilson, Edward O. *Consilience: The Unity of Knowledge.* New York: Vintage Books, 1999.

World Health Organization. Constitution. Geneva: WHO, 1960.

Wright, S.M., J. Daley, E. Peterson, and G.E. Thibault. "Outcomes of Acute Myocardial Infarction in the Department of Veterans Affairs." *Medical Care* 35, no. 2 (1997): 128–41.

Wynia, M.K., D.S. Cummins, J.B. VanGeest, and I.B. Wilson. "Physician Manipulation of Reimbursement Rules for Patients: Between a Rock and a Hard Place." *Journal of the American Medical Association* 283, no. 14 (2000): 1858–65.

Zhang, M. "Physician Case-by-Case Assignment and Participation in Medicare." *Journal of Aging and Social Policy* 9, no. 2 (1997): 19–35.

Zimmerman, R.K., T.A. Mieczjowski, and M. Raymund. "Relationships Between Primary Payer and Use of Proactive Immunization Practices: A National Servey." *American Journal of Managed Care* 5, no. 5 (1999): 574–82.

Index

FEGS

The Downfall of a Non-profit Giant

By Gina P. Thomas

FEGS: THE DOWNFALL OF A NON PROFIT GIANT

Divine Goodness LLC

Waterbury, Connecticut

ISBN -13:978-1979135535

ISBN - 10:1979135533

Printed in the United States of America

Copyright © 2018 Gina P. Thomas

Divine Media

CONTENTS

2

Dedication

To My Heavenly Father who makes all things possible....

To My Lord and Savior, Jesus Christ.

To My Husband for his unconditional love and patience with me.

To My Children, Elijah, Gevonna, Isaiah, Saul, the reason I push.

To Apostle Stan and Pastor Viv, whose prayers have propelled me into this next season.

To Every one of my co-workers at FEGS who withstood this hardship and even walked away with dignity because of the ability you had to endure hardship, I'm grateful to each and every one of you for the years we worked together to service our clients with joy......

FORWARD

Trust is the foundation of any civilized society. It is the foundation of our morals and it is from this level of basic decency that we build communities, we build legacies and we build around us agencies that are designed to garner solutions, agencies that rebuild lives that have been destroyed by societal ills like drugs and incarceration. It is that trust that allows us to help those who cannot help themselves, those who might have lost hope and assist communities build that which plagues them and whatever atrocity they might encounter.

When that trust is broken, when that which is called to do well is blanketed with corruption and deceit, we are no longer civilized. We are then after personal gain and the good of the society is no longer what drives us , we are then consumed with greed and consumption and our morals have become corrupted and we cease to exist.

Chapter 1 The Culture of FEGS

FEGS, formerly known as Federation Employment and Guidance

Service came to a complete halt in 2015 after 80 years of

servicing New York and now everyone had been ordered to get

off the train. For many decades, this powerhouse of an agency

helped clients in more ways than can be imagined, employed

many people and gave them opportunities to gain higher ground

and supported the neighborhoods in which they operated ever

breathing life into the economy. Then like everything that runs

out of life, it died a quick painful death. So many dreams and visions imploding and the lives that FEGS touched, forever changed.

Coming from someone who practically grew with FEGS, I was an employee who loved this agency, I respected the mission and understood how this agency operated, or did I? Did anyone? From the outside looking in, FEGS was a monstrosity that operated with millions of dollars in charitable donations and government monies to provide services to so many sectors of what encompasses the word, need. For every bad thing that happened in the City of New York, FEGS had been given a grant and money to fix it. Remember Gimbels? When they closed in 1987, FEGS received the Dislocated Workers contract to help those out of work, with placement. When Altro closed its doors on Wards Island, FEGS took over the entire building and its workers. When 9/11 happened, FEGS was granted a Mental Health contract to help people through with Mental Health Counseling and the trauma of Terrorism, when the New York Society for the Deaf closed its doors, FEGS was there to overtake them and the workers and lastly, when Hurricane Sandy happened, FEGS received grants to help millions of New Yorkers recover. In between that, were hundreds of contracts, large and small that were in the millions of dollars, and FEGS wanted to and did bid on them all. After all, they had some of the best grant writers, some of the best selling proposal writers in the business, and because FEGS paid handsomely for the higher echelon that was to bring in the money, they flourished, all so that this wonderful agency could remain solvent.

There were two faces to this agency. The one that *appeared* to be successful and did everything by the book and the one that reeked of reality. The reality that FEGS, to some, was a giant cookie jar, an ATM with a few cards issued to those who ran the agency. Few people knew of the reality, the internal workings until it came to the light. Many people thought of FEGS as a corporate entity as opposed to a Non Profit Agency. Management gained notoriety for their efforts in recruiting talent from the best in the business. These efforts on paper, in Request

7

for Proposals, (RFP's), appear necessary and beneficial but were no doubt superfluous, especially considering the outcome as a whole. In doing everyday work, the majority of the workers only thought about the needs of the clients, servicing them to the best of their ability, and engaging clients face to face and at the end f the day, taking home a paycheck. Yet others dealt indirectly through administrative functions, and still others were hired and pegged to oversee the entire workforce at FEGS.

To work for this agency, at one time in history, was an honor and a platform to greater things probably because of the sheer size of the agency and the diversity of its mission. To be hired as a general worker was an exciting process, yet very grueling. I came in 1986 and back at that time, there was fingerprinting, background checks, and the need from the Human Resource department to hire the very best; at least project the image that the employees were the very best. The practice of hiring executives was even more strenuous and the acquisition of Vice President's, Chief Operating Officers and Chief Financial

Officer's came with vetting. When these talents were posted in the New York Not-for- Profit Press, they came with impressive bios that demanded six figure salaries and FEGS was all the willing to pay, even up to its demise. It was in the hands of these top executives to which the Board of Directors entrusted this power house of an agency. After all, collectively, the CEO and the Executive VP had a total of 80 years' experience, the number of years the agency was old. The expectation was so grandiose, that they entrusted their life work and the reputation of the agency to the leadership, to the two who were ultimately responsible for bringing it down.

The façade was phenomenal, even the insiders did not know that this agency was in trouble. Like many, I, my co-workers, the low level managers, the middle managers, the senior managers, some of the executives and the administrators all thought that we would safely retire from this secure agency and live happily ever after. After all, we had seen many of the Executives fly off with golden parachutes. But it appears that no one knew that the ship was sinking. If they did, they certainly did not care. By this time, they were in go for self-mode. The union members had no idea that they were on the way to be bamboozled. Like the majority of workers anywhere, you show up for work to do the job for which you were hired. So long as you get a paycheck at the end of the two weeks, there was no need to question operations.

At the very end, myself and the two other Chapter Chairs of the union for the agency saw that FEGS operated over 300 programs spread across the Bronx, Manhattan, Brooklyn, Queens and Long Island. With all this clout and money they should have been able to salvage programs and cuts should have been clean and seamless. A professional agency with the highest goals, highest expectations one of the highest payouts for Administrators for an agency of this kind should have been building a stronger foundation but instead, they were operating in the 21st Century with a mid-20th century mindset. Operating in a mindset of robbing Peter to pay Paul never really knowing how much was in the cookie jar; just spending and not counting the overhead, the salaries and most importantly, the needs of the clients. During the latter meetings, many of the programs had called in complaining that that they did not even have Personal Needs Allowance to give the clients and basic supplies were dwindling fast. How does this happen? The "workers" were all put into a class by the executives as faithful to the clients, but mindless…."they only know what we tell them and for the most part, believe everything that we tell them". There had been growing dissension among the rank and file membership that Executive Management had become increasingly callous of the needs of the members. All of this came to a head and while there was plenty of blame to go around, we the membership should not really have been surprised. We always knew that there was a disparity but no one really questioned the finances. We thought FEGS had deep, deep pockets but more importantly we believed that FEGS was fiscally responsible.

I came to FEGS during its heyday and found this agency to be of the highest caliber in everything that they did. I came from a grassroots organization in the Northwest Bronx and was hired to work in downtown Manhattan. At 25 years old, and no real knowledge of anything big, I was excited to say the least, to be a part of what I saw as the corporations of the non-profits. At the helm at this time was a genius. Al Miller, one who had risen through the ranks to become a CEO for this high ranking organization and was certainly capable of taking this agency to higher heights. FEGS started as FES in 1934, a mission for Jewish Immigrants who were finding it hard to find employment during and after the Great Depression. The agency at this time was being funded by wealthy Jewish Philanthropies to help those in need.

As the funding increased, so did the span of services and by the time I came in 1986, Federation, Employment and Guidance Service had become so much more than employment, They had a Trades and Business School, Day Habilitation programs for the severely mentally handicapped, Residential Services for those with severe developmental disabilities and programs for inmates and ex-offenders. They had educational programs for youth and had been selected to pilot programs in the shelter and responding to the closures of the States Mental hospitals, FEGS had taken on housing and providing program services for this population. They had more Article 31 clinics and Article 16 clinics than any hospital in the area. They were like Pac Man. Taking on projects, writing dynamic proposals, and because they had space everywhere, managed to operate well and do some very wonderful things. It was quite impressive to see this behemoth of an agency in operation.

I began my mission as an OJT Employment Specialist, Working with the best counselor there was. I had my own office and went from servicing just two small classrooms of teens in the Bronx, at a local grassroots organization to servicing what seemed like everyone who was seeking a job in Manhattan. I was accustomed to the small and mundane, I went from developing my own jobs to watching a team of Account Managers develop jobs, sector specific for the people whom we had to place in employment. Yes, FEGS was a machine and Al Miller was the captain. As the agency was structured like a hierarchy, the union workers were on the bottom underneath a long chain of command. During this time, it was okay for FEGS to operate in such a manner because overhead was not as costly, space could be shared, and more money was flowing and people liked and trusted non- profits. They liked and trusted FEGS. They were do-gooders with missions to help those around them and make the neighborhoods better places to live. Almost everyone in New York knew of FEGS and knew of a FEGS program that was nearby. An agency that was interwoven in the fabric of almost every neighborhood in the boroughs.

More importantly, these were professionals at the top of their game passing on their expertise to those coming in and teaching the newcomers how a not for profit operates. Smaller non-profits came to FEGS for training on how to operate, how to better service clients and mushroom into to a full service smorgasbord. I remember the leadership of the previous agency for which I worked coming to training at FEGS and asking me, "What are you doing here?" My response was proudly, "I work here". What a feeling. I was apart of something big, with my eyes set on growing with the agency and learning all that I could about my position and passing on this expertise to others looking for employment as well as any other function that commandeered this agency.

Internally and at the top, Al Miller was developing a team that would take this agency to the next level and even global. We were reasonably kept abreast of what was going on in the agency but never knew of all the fund raisers, charitable donations and monies that were allotted to FEGS. Right by Al Miller's side was Ira Machowsky, someone who also had risen to the ranks and was slated to take the helm as CEO when FEGS imploded. Ira had a plaque in his office which read that he was the "Chief

Cornerstone of FEGS". This is a well know scripture in the Bible which states that Jesus is the Chief Cornerstone. A corner stone does not become undone, so I guess the former was not the real thing.

As time went on, Ira grew in rank and when Al Miller retired in 2007, I'm sure he believed that he was leaving FEGS in good hands with Gail Magiliff as CEO and Ira Machowsky as Executive Vice President and if you know the culture of FEGS, Ira was really in charge. Truth be told, no one really knew Gail's role. We knew her title, but her role was one of coming into meetings with her infamous purse to make small or big talk and tell of all the wonderful things FEGS was doing. New collaborations, seamless merging and watching the budget.

So what happened, why did this happen? And who was to blame? It certainly was not the staff who diligently came to work every day to provide what was needed and required for the clients. Clients depended on the services that FEGS rendered and workers, although moderately paid, gave their all. Many

16

workers knew that FEGS was not a gravy train but it was at least

safe and secure. At least, we knew that we would be getting paid

every two weeks.   It was well known that the salary gap at

FEGS ranged from $22,000 for our lowest paid union employees

to $427,700, Nathan-kazis, J. (2015, September 15). FEGS Execs got fat Payouts as

Bankruptcy Loomed Amid Rampant Mismanagement. Retrieved April 18, 2018, a base

salary for Gail Magiliff, the CEO who commanded this salary at

the time FEGS went belly up. What kind of disparity is that?

These were the basis for the arguments between the union and

management throughout negotiations. The union's voice was

loud and boisterous against this type of salary differences and

gave impact statements that clearly illustrated the difficulties

people on staff were having paying rent, buying food and

keeping up with bare necessities while management shook their

heads and looked at us and stated that they understood how hard

it was for their staff. Gail would come back with lines like "We

certainly know the difficulties you are having and we can

certainly relate". How could Ira relate when he had a bi-weekly salary of $14, 004.04, Nathan-kazis, J. (2015, September 15).

FEGS Execs got fat Payouts as Bankruptcy Loomed Amid

Rampant Mismanagement. Retrieved April 18, 2018. Really!

Union employees would be furious at their treatment by the

Executives but fighting them was a collective effort. As I write

this, I have to marvel at their condescending tone and audacity

that would they would even insult us as they did. Union

employees who were fortunate enough to sit on the negotiation

teams resounded with their discontent, but it all fell on deaf ears.

How does someone who is making $400,000 understand about

an employee's inability to pay a bill, someone's homelessness or

the need for an employee to borrow from the agency's loan fund?

Many of the union employees needed to take advantage of this

program including myself. Even Ira Machowky who was

making a not so shabby $343,000 Nathan-kazis, J. (2015,

September 15). FEGS Execs got fat Payouts as Bankruptcy

Loomed Amid Rampant Mismanagement. Retrieved April 18,

2018, would chime in and lead the charge that the agency had a "fiscal responsibility" to ensure that the agency remained sound and solvent.

But this was the culture of FEGS. To pay the executives exorbitant salaries, while the workers scrambled to make it from paycheck to paycheck. I clearly understand that the higher you go on the totem pole and the more you oversee, the higher your salary should be. But this was not a corporation operating in the private sector. It was supposed to be a not - for - profit agency. Although FEGS did invest in some private holdings and set up external operations to manage what was done on the inside, and it was running these operations as corporations that   was responsible for ultimately signing their death warrant. Much of the problem stemmed from the agency's attempt to conduct profit making ventures. All Sector, an FEGS subsidiary, born as the "synergy" of not-for-profit and for profit business, in 1998 was the brainchild of Al Miller and others to add a profit making business to an already lucrative agency. The idea of course was to make money and I'm sure that top heads approached this as a means of investing and hopefully make a killing in profits since IT was always seen as a money maker. The problem with this is that you are not playing with your own money. If they were, then the agency would not have had to eat the 72 million dollars in losses that All Sector garnered during its 16 years in operations.

Chapter 2 The Union

Many might ask, on whose authority am I able to write this. Anyone who knew me at FEGS knew that I had been at this agency a very long time and had gotten to know many people from all sides of the fence, the Union, Human Resources and Management. I had garnered many relationships because I worked well with my coworkers and worked equally as hard on behalf of them if they had been in any trouble during their tenure at FEGS. I worked with, as part of a team, union leaders who also knew very well the agency for which they worked. I studied the contracts, help formulate some of the changes, attended many conventions to assimilate changes in laws that would affect nonprofits, but most importantly, I was a worker an everyday worker who had diversified my work portfolio by applying to

21

and working for many programs throughout the agency. I had gone from Employment Counseling to Job Development to Training to Facilitating workshops for inmates on Rikers Island to Case Management in Mental Health. These experiences helped me to see the agency from many different lenses. Actively involving myself in the union at first as Shop Steward , then Chief Steward only capped the knowledge I had attained and broadened my horizons as to what I was able to do for myself and more importantly really go in and help and assist others.

The union was a collective effort, an arm of the District Council 1707, Local 215. Those union employees working in leadership positions were all long term employees who knew FEGS well. We developed a rapport with Human Resource Dynamic (HRD) and in many cases sought to and actually averted terminations and helped in what we felt were unfair disciplines and decisions.

I was a part of the union. I was hired into a position that was project and unionized. I was hired at $18,900 in a Master's level position. Because of my experience and a Bachelor's Degree, I was a sure fit. I didn't know too much about the union except that I had to pay dues every month and the person whose place I took was a Shop Steward. What was that? The Shop Steward was someone who advocated for the workers in their shop. Someone who might be the eyes and ears of the workplace.

As I continued to work, I liked the world I had entered and because of how FEGS spaced their programs, I was on the floor with a diverse group of people performing all types of functions for the agency. The Chief Steward at the time was a nurse, but she also was the Chapter Chair of the agency. The Chapter Chair is the Chief Shop Steward who oversees the union activity for the agency. They are responsible for representing workers in grievances, disciplinary hearings, arbitration hearings and they are to ensure that agency is abiding by the union contract.

FEGS' contract was with DC1707, Local 215 AFSCME, which was the union for nonprofits and specifically under Local 215, a division for Social Services agencies. I was being recruited by The Union Chapter Chair to attend union meetings just to see how they operated. At this time of my life, I was like a sponge, ever learning and wanting to learn about what I was doing and finding out what type of agency it was for which I worked. It was fascinating and soon after, I was asked to sit on my first negotiating team. I also attended classes at Cornell Labor University to learn as much as I could about Unions, Grievances and the process of Collective Bargaining. I had attended various conferences and learned an endless amount about unions and how they operated, how management was always going to be on one side and union on another. These thought processes were where I started, not where I ended.

Sitting across from management for the first time was intimidating, I didn't know if I could freely speak or would I be judged based on who I was and the position I was in. Well I thought that I would watch and take over from there. I appreciated the revelations that were shared in Human Resources (HRD) and how this was a "perfect agency" that never made a mistake and the union members were watched and evaluated on the standards of near perfection. It took years to learn that workers were hired not to make mistakes. This was the FEGS culture. It always took pleading on their behalf to give employees another chance or look at the mitigating circumstances surrounding the events that seemed to pop up almost on a daily basis.

FEGS always felt the need to separate themselves from anything and anyone that would cause controversy or make them look less than excellent... This was always conflicting because the union members, it seemed should never make a mistake. If they did, they were demonized. They were held to a different standard than management and no matter how obvious this was, management was believed in their reporting of an incident more often than the union. There was divisiveness but many employees were intimidated and never wanted to openly complain. There were times when I would observe managers coming to work late and strolling in way past the work day and the excuse from HRD would be that we did not know if the manager was coming from a meeting or anyplace else. Yeah right! The work day started at 8:30 am for most and the manager is strolling into the food court at 8:50 am. What meeting transpired from their walk from the train to the coffee shop? These disparities caused hostility at times and at times the union was accused of not doing enough. This was not the case. We were just not getting the responses that we wanted from HRD.

FEGS prided itself in the way that they operated. They looked for ways in which to measure their own standards. So an organization like CARF (Commission on Accreditation of Rehabilitation facilities), which was the highest accreditation that an agency could have, was always a triennial goal. Audits were constantly done; quality assurance became a regular department and Inspector Generals who investigated malfecenses committed by the workers, sat in judgment of staff based on Compliance standards created by New York State. The union saw so many people lose their jobs, get disciplined because the standards always reiterated at a disciplinary hearing or grievance meeting was to insure that no one did anything that would jeopardize the integrity of FEGS. No one should be able to minimize the quality that the agency set for itself. I almost believed that those in the Executive Position did absolutely nothing wrong. I even marveled how the executives would say that they did not call in sick, almost creating in the unionized employees a wall of shame if they dared to do anything contrary to that. But looking back on some of the reasons people were terminated have paled in comparison to making an agency implode and had one of our union employees been responsible for the implosion, they probably would be serving time at ADMAX , The Federal Maximum Prison in Florence Colorado.

For argument sake, no I do not believe the demise of the agency was an intentional thing but paying forward to Executives 93,000, 75,000, 50,000 respectively as you are headed out the door and putting in for and receiving a 35,000 vacation payout and the agency had just announced that they were $20 million in the hole, to me *is* criminal, intentional and egregious. To further deny workers their severance that they were entitled to after so many years of service , to deny them vacation and then move to file bankruptcy so that we would have an even more difficult time receiving monies that are owed to us is barbaric, inhumane and illustrates the way we really were viewed. The sad commentary is that this disgusting behavior was not just implemented to the union staff, many of the low level managers, middle managers and even senior managers were force fed garbage and ended up without any oars in their boats. They were screaming for lifeboats but were given none. They too had been bamboozled. Where was their money, their severance and vacation? To add insult to injury, they had no union which to file a lawsuit to receive their monies in any timely fashion and from the looks as to the picture as a whole, some of them might not ever see the totality of their money.

All of these nuances in some way shape an agency to a pattern of thinking and that pattern of thinking was played all the way to the bank. The agency would reek of money. In the first negotiations in which I participated, I sat across from men and women who resembled the Wall Street Corporate Executives of JP Morgan, Goldman Sachs and there were attorneys who were actually from Proskauer and Rose. The plea on behalf of their agency was simple. Federation Employment and Guidance Service as it was referred to back then, was so prideful on how they got the job done. "We truly appreciate all that you do" (referring to all the union workers). But your hard work, your degrees, your expertise, your rapport with our clients could really never be paid for. We have **this** amount of money for *you* and nothing more. In developing and shaping the union contracts that went forth then continued over the years, the union was always told what they wanted us to believe. There were times, especially early on, that we were able to negotiate a little more, but the ceiling of the final amount was never really presented. This was something for which we had to push. We even had job actions and in some years, we came very close to a strike. Some of the managers never saw what we experienced, especially during the times of the negotiations. We were privy to arrogance at times, we were told that we didn't understand the business side, we were not contending with the economy, as if we as the union members, were living in a bubble. We knew first hand of what it was like living paycheck to paycheck. Many managers were advised of these negotiations but always thought that the unions' need to protect its members were exaggerated and we as union reps were overzealous angry workers who really hated management. This was not the case. We did know however, the truth. We knew some things about the executives that other managers knew nothing about.

We as the union did our research as to how much money did FEGS really have and how much of that pie went to overhead, services, clients, staff and management. When I first began at FEGS, there was a mantra on all our cards, placards and stationary which proudly displayed that "FEGS charged no fees for our services". That meant something. As time progressed, that mantra was replaced for solicitation of donations and being reimbursed for everything that they provided. UJA, a very prominent agency that assisted FEGS in raising money and giving matching grants and funding was on their stationary and to most of the union staff symbolized money. Prior to the negotiations, we would view the tax form 990 to eye the salaries of the top executives and from the very beginning, we, the union and other staff always believed that the Executives of FEGS made way too much money but it really was never questioned, *obviously*, because FEGS delivered on all the contracts it had with the city and made good on completing the goals of the RFP's, (request for proposals) mainly because of the excellent work of the staff it employed. Despite the implosion, the union worked diligently to balance what they had to work with and keep as many people as possible employed as it could.

Chapter 3 The Management

Management at FEGS was multi-tiered. This system was put in place because the agency had a relatively strong and active union. So management felt the need to counter this intelligence with levels upon levels of management. It was the Executive Management's way of ensuring that they had the upper hand on the staff that they employed.

There were low level supervisors, middle management who were in charge of overseeing the many programs FEGS operated, senior managers and the Executives who ultimately and literally drove FEGS into the ground without remorse and without a true assessment of the damage that was caused because of power and greed. It's similar to running someone over with a vehicle and not stopping or even looking back in the rear views to see or care for that person you hit.

The Senior Executives somehow believed that they had absolute autonomy. All power and every decision was theirs to make concerning the business of the agency. Material for which a good drama is made or a best selling reality show. A year and a half later, the workers and clients are still feeling the ripple effect of poor management, greed and the illusion that we, the workers and the clients meant so much to an agency that went to great

lengths to provide golden parachutes for their executives.

At the time of the implosion, the CEO, Gail Magaliff was

making $435,000 more than the President of the United States,

and she certainly was not working to that capacity but this is

human service dollars we are talking about, government monies,

charity, all donated and given on the basis that there is a

designated population that will be serviced and their collective

needs will be met. Somehow when a budget was done at the end

of the fiscal year, executives included their astronomical salaries

without a blink. Even prior to them closing their programs and

shuttering the door for good, as indicated earlier, as Ira

Machowsky gave himself upwards of $93,000 as a bonus and

distributed, I guess according to camaraderie, bonuses to other

executives so that their pockets and bank accounts could be

lined and padded. This is dereliction of duty and it speaks to the

need for not for profit reform on so many levels. When the

smoke cleared, the Board of Directors began to see the light and recommended or accepted two key resignations, the two aforementioned executives. Many questions lingered. Did anyone on the board question the final amount given to these executives as they were going out the door? Which leads to another question, who was on the board and what was their allegiance to the two top Executives FEGS employed? The responsibility of a Board of Directors is to oversee the company's affairs and ensure that the company, agency in this case, prosper according to the mission and stated goals and oversee allocated funds in order to stay afloat. They were asleep at the wheel.

Why were people given five figure bonuses? When it was disclosed that there was a 20 million dollar deficit? This begs the question, who on the Board was getting paid and what were they being paid?

As the union contract was being negotiated, did anyone not see this when they were doing projected budgets? They issued to the entire negotiating team a PowerPoint presentation outlining their budget and how much money they had as an agency and where they saw themselves going form 2015-2018. What an absolute joke. An analysis or a simple forecast would have shown them that they were heading for an iceberg. We are talking about very intelligent people who at the very appearance, you automatically assume they got it going on!

In looking back, I believe that they were not as smart as they appeared. They did not stay to answer any questions. They did not believe that they owed us that much. Union members were traumatized and directed their questions to the union, who was equally dumbfounded

No one could answer any questions. As the Chapter Chair, people were calling me off the wall to find out what was going on. We were all standing around by our cubicles wondering what was happening and how was this all going to pan out. No one had any answers. Especially since we had successfully negotiated a new union contract six - months prior and were expected to be looking at raises coming in a few months. How was this all going to be possible? Was this the biggest long con job in history, (like those bank jobs that set off a sense of notoriety) or was the CFO of FEGS that oblivious or was she being paid to write reports that were not true. All I know is 2+2=4. 2+2 does not equal 400,000. There were three CFO's hired in three years. The first one must have hauled out after he saw the condition of the books. Prior to him coming on, Leonard Silver had been in that position. What was he doing all that time? He would always have one hand over his mouth and his eyes would always be squinting as if he knew something we didn't and he was trying to determine if we should know or not.

This type of deficit does not pop up overnight. Even if Mr. Silver had been gone for three years, was there any evidence that the agency was even in a hint of trouble? The agency felt the need to continue to do things the way that they have been doing things for years.

When you look at an agency's books, you have to look back. Who was monitoring the $250 million that was coming to the agency annually?

A meeting was held with the new CEO, and other executives as well as with union leadership and an Excel presentation was delivered and we were looking at figures with a bunch of numbers all going in the wrong direction and the words FEGS is insolvent ringing in our ears like church bells on an organ at a public funeral. I sat there and watched them play out three scenarios of what would happen if they kept FEGS open and how the finances would look three years later. It was a disaster. Even I, one who is not proficient at math, could see the hole FEGS had dug and even if they looked at their finances for two or three years back, they would have seen the titanic coming at us and all they had to do was turn the wheel. Yet only going two years back the Senior Management had hired two CFO's, one COO, and one Administrative Vice President. These titles with bodies did not come cheap. In developing a projected budget, they had

38

to know this would implode. I don't know whether it was pride, them thinking, "How far can we take this?" "How long can we ride this gravy train? No we don't know anyone's thoughts and intentions; we do know that there is a level of accountability of those at the top and their responsibility to their subordinates.

From an analytical point of view, the Executives have a moral obligation to ensure that all finances were accounted for and budgets balanced. In management's presentation to the union, they indicated that FEGS management failed to upgrade their financial system and the way they were doing their booking was sorely outdated and had not been keeping up with the times This seemed to be obtuse. This statement is justified by the modernization of the entire agency, new fleet of vehicles, the computer programs and equipment was updated, modernized decor, security upgrades and even the newer accommodations as a result of Medicaid reimbursements as the conversion was made to Managed Care. How does an agency take special care to ensure that it operates with state of the art equipment, then align itself with the best in the business but fail to upgrade its financial system to the point where a 20 million dollar deficit is not visible on any computer and no one notices or fails to sound the alarm?

You can use the excuse that they used with the union during union negotiations and sit across from us and declare that they have no money that they are on the "brink of collapse". This certainly was not the fault of the clients, nor was this the fault of the workers. They had the brightest of the brightest when it came to talent acquisition as they sought CFO after CFO to come in and clean up the mess that they had made. It would be like what happened in the banking industry in 2008. The culmination of all of the above played some part in the agency's downfall and bigwigs who could no longer fake the farce that ultimately affected thousands of lives. As a matter of fact, all those who lived through this ordeal will never be the same.

Chapter 4 The Clients

The clients of FEGS were absolutely devastated to hear that the agency that they depended upon had shuttered their doors. After all, it was always the needs of clients that precipitated a need for an agency to provide those services. In the very beginning, FES

41

developed goals and programs around the needs of the clients. They would never have expected to be paid for providing this service. After all, helping other Jewish Immigrants settle in by ensuring that they ascertain employment was a priority and a privilege. Even in my early years at the agency, the mantra, "We charge no fees for our services" was plastered everywhere and any one taking advantage of this was dealt with harshly.

Think about it, why should any fees be associated with a not for profit agency whose primary goal is to help the many needs of the clients in the community? Why charge fees when sectors of the government was providing millions of dollars to get these services done? The truth be told, as FES evolved into Federation Employment and Guidance Service, the expectations became a little more and the dynamics of a once simple agency became ever more complex. New leadership brought with it a new vision. A genius and well known in the not for profit private sector community, Al Miller, the CEO did remarkable things in his heyday with the organization which allowed FEGS to grow and prosper to the conglomerate it was ultimately known. The driving force was not always greed. It was an organization with a humane mission that sought to genuinely care for the needs of the people in the New York City communities. The client pool began to grow with the changes in laws and the implementation of various legislative mandates. For example, the closing of the state Mental Health facilities created a vast need for housing of the mentally ill and the developmentally disabled. FEGS was not only willing to take on this population but they had the facilities to undertake this massive endeavor. They worked tirelessly with regulatory agencies in order to put these visions into actions and ultimately. FEGS was prospering like no other agency of its kind.

Of the three groups of people, the most vulnerable were the clients. They came to, were assigned to, and referred to the agency based on a need. Some of them were so severely disabled that even the knowledge of who FEGS was escaped them. To those who were more cognizant of their surroundings, this was their daily bread. The need base was phenomenal. As the

funding continued to grow, the more varied was the services and

to the very end, FEGS kept the hiring farce going establishing

that they needed these top level people to manage this animal

that somehow grew out of control. For example, why would

you hire three Chief Financial Officers in the last three years of

the life of the agency? Was there something to hide? Were each

of the CFO's unable to rectify the mess that already was or was

the undertaking so big, that for those looking at the depth of

chaos and confusion in the finances, that they refused to do this

and fled. At one of the latter meetings with the Union

Delegation and some Senior Managers who had decided to tend

to FEGS' end of Life care, the reveal of the financial analysis

was that FEGS was operating an antiquated system that had not

been upgraded with the times. They were still doing things by

hand. In the world of numbers, it doesn't take a genius to figure

out that all the upgrades in monetary contributions required an upgraded system that needed to be precise and be able to document penny by penny.

Many of the workers did remarkable jobs dedicating their lives to an agency with a mission, oblivious to the fact that there was trouble brewing from another angle. The clients of this agency were just as uninformed, their caregivers went on their daily routine believing that FEGS would go into the history books as one of the largest agencies of its kind. The clients were unsuspecting, even those just seeking employment, took this as some temporary problem that could be fixed with some type of wand, this was not the case. The suffering was real and no one was spared.

Chapter 5 Where do we go from here?

How do you move on from this place? As one who has been affected, my life has been forever changed. Not because I could not find another place of employment nor because I was not qualified, rather, I just was not prepared. When you set goals and believe that you are going to retire from an agency or job, you kind of settle in. Most of the employees of FEGS were long termers or lifers if you will, simply because of the stability that the agency, almost guaranteed. They had built so many models of examples and this indicated that this agency was going to be around for the long haul.

Many former employees fell sick or were too sick at the time of the demise that panic set in because of their medical needs. From the time of the notification that the agency was not solvent, the Executives in place began dismantling the agency and someone who had been in employed for twenty nine years by this one agency, had less than two months before I was put out, evicted, from my place of employment.

I had no time to plan, no time to even look for a job. I was facing unemployment and a dismal outlook. While we, the union were fighting for the workers, time was not on our side and those WARN (Worker Adjustment and Retraining notification) notifications had gone out, (this was an act requiring certain

47

employers to notify their employee in advance in the event of a mass lay off) but not timely, so many contracts had been breached, but no one cared, not about me, my coworkers, my supervisor, my director and most importantly, the clients. The goal was now to get us out as quickly as possible and without delay.

Many of the clients were confused as they were not fully aware of where they would end up and some did not have the level of understanding to comprehend the magnitude of what had just happened. They went from total dependency to being shoved away from their life support system. Even though other agencies were pegged to take over, clients thrive with stability and just knowing that they did not have the workers who had been with them for twenty and thirty years was devastating to say the least.

I was interviewed by a New York Times Photojournalist who was doing a human interest story as to how an agency with the clout that FEGS once held, and have been around so long and had impacted the workers and the clients and community like they did, fall. They wanted to know how I felt about their actions. All I could say was that I was so in shock and hurt by what had been done that I really felt betrayed. I also, at that time, did not know what was in store for me. There I was with a mortgage, car note and bills and no job.

Where was an agency to help those of us who were seeking some relief...? All the money that had been taken in by FEGS and there was nothing for us. They did not want to give us our vacation or severance pay and shortly after all the inquiries came rolling in about money, they filed for bankruptcy. The plan was to get out of their obligation to the people who had dedicated half their lives to an agency that dropped them like a hot potato. This type of behavior, was so cruel and calculating. Even at the meeting, the previous administration had hurriedly made an exit. Neither the CEO nor Executive Vice President offered to sit with the people that they had worked with for so many years and explain what had happened. This is what made it so suspicious. When you have people who have worked for the agency for so many years and leave within one day of speaking with you indicates to me that there was something to hide and you want to get far away from the impending danger.

So many questions, to this day, that have still not been answered. The sting somehow always comes back to take a pinch at the core of your soul. To not understand fully brings to the forefront our need as human beings to have closure in any given situation and this never happened. Of course you move on, you reestablish, you find other employment and you ultimately go on with your life. Many had no choice but to take this path. For others, it has not been that easy. Some have landed other employment that did not last, some were not able to even do that.

I'm sure many therapists are cashing in on the lost tribe of FEGS because their future has been so uncertain and the exit has caused Post Traumatic Stress Disorder in many and any thread of human decency has turned into anger and mistrust. The former workers of FEGS have formed a Facebook page to support one another and work with each other towards finding employment

50

and helping each other get through what still manages to spark a chord in anyone who did work for FEGS.

To this day, some of the union workers did get a portion of their severance pay in 2016 and the management and administrative staff just receive theirs in 2017 with both sectors still trying to get vacation pay that is owed to them. The Bankruptcy matter is still in court with other vendors seeking relief from an agency whose Executives have long packed up and moved on.

These actions beg for reform in the not for profit world and better guidelines and stipulations which would not allow those that use public money for their own gain to go without prosecution. Even if the very appearance finds that no law was broken, no Executive should be able to walk away with money that rightfully was awarded by the city or state or even private funding, These monies should be earmarked accordingly and the use of that money should not be readily available like an ATM for those looking for a path to wealth that they did not earn.

Bibliography

Nathan-kazis, J. (2015, September 15). FEGS Execs got fat Payouts as

Bankruptcy Loomed Amid Rampant Mismanagement. Retrieved April 18,

2018.

Made in the USA
Middletown, DE
20 January 2023

22641423R00033